MODERNISING HEALTH CARE

Reinventing professions, the state and the public

Ellen Kuhlmann

First published in Great Britain in September 2006 by

The Policy Press
University of Bristol
Fourth Floor
Beacon House
Queen's Road
Bristol BS8 1QU
UK

Tel +44 (0)117 331 4054
Fax +44 (0)117 331 4093
e-mail tpp-info@bristol.ac.uk
www.policypress.org.uk

© Ellen Kuhlmann 2006

British Library Cataloguing in Publication Data
A catalogue record for this book is available from the British Library.

Library of Congress Cataloging-in-Publication Data
A catalog record for this book has been requested.

ISBN-10 1 86134 858 4 hardcover
ISBN-13 978 1 86134 858 6 hardcover

Ellen Kuhlmann researches and teaches at the Centre for Social Policy Research at the University of Bremen, Germany.

Cover design by Qube Design Associates, Bristol.
Printed and bound by CPI Group (UK) Ltd, Croydon, CR0 4YY

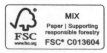

MIX
Paper | Supporting
responsible forestry
FSC
www.fsc.org
FSC® C013604

Contents

List of tables and figures

Tables

Figures

Acknowledgements

I would like to express my thanks to those who have contributed in different ways to this work. A grant from the University of Bremen (ZF/27/820/1) allowed me to do the research and work on the book. The Statutory Health Insurance (SHI) Physicians' Associations North Rhine and Westphalia-Lippe and the Physicians' Chamber North Rhine supported a questionnaire study of office-based physicians. Other professional associations helped me to gather primary material and organise focus group discussions and expert interviews, namely the Physicians' Chamber Bremen, and the Federal and Regional Associations of Physiotherapists and Surgery Receptionists. Rolf Müller carried out statistical analysis; Maren Stamer assisted with the organisation of focus groups with patients from self-help groups and collected additional expert interviews in 2005; and Nadine Helwig, Oda von Rhaden and Brunhild Schröder contributed as students to the project. Angela Rast-Margerison, with her usual patience and proficiency, translated parts of the book and edited the full typescript; she helped to maintain confidence that my writing will turn out as an English typescript. I am also grateful to the numerous participants in the study.

Numerous colleagues from the Research Network 'Sociology of Professions' of the European Sociological Association, and the Research Committee 'Professional Groups' of the International Sociological Associations, as well as the audience of other international meetings on the professions, health care and social policy, provided the opportunity to discuss my research in its early stages and helped to sharpen my theoretical arguments. My special thanks go to those who commented on papers or draft chapters or otherwise collaborated during the research process and encouraged me to bring the German case of modernising health care into an international debate; in particular, Judith Allsop, Birgit Blättel-Mink, Celia Davies, Julia Evetts, Gerd Glaeske, Karin Gottschall, Michael Hülsmann, Petra Kolip and Mike Saks. I owe a great deal to Viola Burau for bringing me closer to social policy and comparative approaches and for her inspiring comments on the draft typescript, and to Janet Newman, who supported my ideas at a crucial point in the writing and invited me to The Open University. And finally, many thanks to the team at The Policy Press for their kindness and support during the publication process.

Abbreviations

CAM	complementary and alternative medicine
CHD	coronary heart disease
CNM	certified nurse midwife
DMP	disease management programme
EBM	evidence-based medicine
EU	European Union
GMC	General Medical Council
GP	general practitioner
HEDIS	Health Plan Employer Data and Information Set
HMO	health maintenance organisation
IoM	Institute of Medicine
MCO	managed care organisation
NGO	non-governmental organisation
NHS	National Health Service (Britain)
NP	nurse practitioner
NPM	new public management
PA	physician's assistant
PCG	primary care group
PCT	primary care trust
RCT	randomised controlled trial
SHI	Statutory Health Insurance
WHO	World Health Organization

Glossary

Ambulatory care (*Ambulante Versorgung*)
Health care provided outside the hospitals by office-based generalists and specialists in Germany

Disease management programmes (DMPs)
New models of ambulatory care in Germany that focus on certain chronic illnesses: coronary heart disease (CHD), diabetes mellitus and breast cancer

General (medical) care (*Hausärztliche Versorgung*)
In the German context the term refers to care provided by four types of office-based generalists (*Hausärzte*): physicians specialised in general medicine; physicians who provide general medical care without specialisation (*Praktische Ärzte*); physicians specialised in internal medicine who have to opt for either general care or specialist care; paediatricians are also partly included

General practitioners (GPs)
Physicians who provide general medical care in countries with a gatekeeper system

German gatekeeper model (*Hausarztmodelle*)
Pilot projects aimed at targeting ambulatory care in Germany through a gatekeeper model of office-based generalists; participation is voluntary and open to those who provide general care

Health occupations
In the German context the term refers to all health care workers who are not members of the self-regulating professions (physicians, dentists)

Health professions
Used in the German context the term refers to the classic professions, particularly physicians; used in an international context it comprises all qualified health care workers

Modernisation/late modernity
Used to host broader developments and transformations in various areas of societies, that is, changing modes of citizenship, without applying 'grand narratives' of 'late' or 'post'-modernity or 'never have been modern'; with this respect, 'late modernity' refers to features of 21st-century societies that are in some respect different from earlier times

New governance
> Refers to a complex set of regulatory mechanisms and more hybrid patterns that go beyond hierarchical institutional regulation (performance)

Office-based physicians
> Physicians who provide ambulatory care in Germany, comprising generalists and specialists

Primary care
> Refers to multidisciplinary caring models in Anglo–American countries according to the World Health Organization (WHO) definition

Professional autonomy
> Used as a normative term related to the claims of professions on self-determination

Social Code Book V (*Sozialgesetzbuch V*)
> Legal framework basically regulating statutory health insurance and health care in Germany

Statutory Health Insurance (SHI) funds/sickness funds (*Gesetzliche Krankenkassen*)
> Non-profit health insurance funds with mandatory membership of approximately 90% of the citizens; together with physicians' associations they form the core of joint self-administration of SHI health care in Germany

User/consumer/patient
> 'User' marks a position in relation to providers and avoids normative distinctions;'consumer'/'consumerism' refers to a political discourse of users as stakeholders;'patient' refers to the micro-level of provider–user relationship and a medical discourse of user participation

Introduction

Health care is a key arena of the modernisation of welfare states. Tighter resources and a changing spectrum of diseases, coupled with new modes of citizenship and demands for public safety, challenge the health care systems throughout the Western world. This book sets out to examine new perspectives on the governance of health care and to highlight the role of the professions as mediators between the state and its citizens. It brings the interdependence and tensions between the health professions, the state and public interest into focus that release ongoing dynamics into the health system. The emerging patterns of a new professionalism in late modernity and interprofessional dynamics lie at the centre of my investigation.

I have chosen the German health care system, and in particular ambulatory care, as a case study to place this national restructuring in the context of European health systems and global reform models. I have applied a multidisciplinary approach that links the study of professions to social policy and health care research. My empirical research takes into account the provider and the user perspective, and a gendered division of the health workforce. Investigating the dynamics of new modes of governance in a non-Anglo-American context of corporatist stakeholder regulation expands the scope of health policy and makes new options apparent that move beyond marketisation and managerialism. The book highlights the context-dependency of medical power and the significance of regulatory frameworks in targeting the rise of a more inclusive professionalism. It helps to clarify whether and how new governance creates 'citizen professionals' that better serve 21st-century societies' health care needs and wants of a diverse public.

Understanding the dynamics of new governance in health care

Health care is being modernised around the Western world. New models of governance have been introduced to reduce medical power and to advance an integrated health workforce and the participation of users. These developments are part of broader changes in the public sector and society at large. They can be explained in terms of modernisation processes that are related to changing modes of citizenship and new models of governance. The restructuring of health care mirrors 'new directions in social policy' (Clarke, 2004) and a move away from hierarchical institutional regulation towards more flexible and hybrid patterns of governing 'peoples and the public sphere' (Newman, 2005a). At the same time, "health care politics are more than a subset of welfare politics and the health care state is more than a subsystem of the welfare state" (Moran, 1999, p 4). The 'meeting' of changing welfare states and changes emanating from the health care system and the health professions need further investigation; controversy remains especially as to whether new governance actually shifts the balance of power away from the medical profession, and which model of provider organisation serves best to improve the accountability of professionals.

In all countries cost containment is a strong policy driver, and marketisation and managerialism are the uncontested 'favourites' of policy makers. "Reform has become a way of life for health services, not only in the UK, but throughout the western world" (Annandale et al, 2004, p 1; see Blank and Burau, 2004; Dubois et al, 2006). However, to date, neither the potential for nor obstacles to change have been investigated in a non-Anglo-American context. Strategies are developed against a backdrop of Anglo-American health systems but new terms are travelling around the world as part of a global discourse on reform. Globalisation and the European unification reinforce the tensions between global models of regulation and provider organisation, and local conditions, needs and demands on health care.

Germany fits the typology of neither market-driven nor state-centred restructuring; it has its one strong and long-lasting tradition of social policy, and the longest tradition of compulsory social health insurance (Greß et al, 2004). While Bismarckian social policy, especially health care, marked a model of social security and justice for about a century, the corporatist structure is nowadays viewed as a barrier to innovation. At the same time, elements of corporatism and professional self-regulation allow for flexibility and responsiveness and may 'buffer' social conflict (Stacey, 1992); they are even gaining ground in state-centred health systems (Allsop, 1999). Transformations of the corporatist system of stakeholder regulation thus provide the opportunity to study both weaknesses and benefits of medical self-regulation. Placing developments in the German health system in a global context of health care restructuring helps to better understand how regulatory frameworks shape and reshape medical power, and brings into focus new health policy options.

A further contribution of this study to the debate on governing health care is its focus on the professions. This approach moves beyond institutional regulation and brings into view reflexivity of change and different sets of dynamics. I argue that professions are key players in health care and mediators between states and citizens. Each side needs the other, and intersections and tensions of interest are therefore inevitably embedded in the triangle comprising health professions, the state and the public. New patterns of governance and new demands on health care challenge the health professions, but in various ways that are not fully under control of governments. Professionalism has the capacity to remake itself and ensure professional power under conditions of changing welfare states and new demands on health care services.

However, the varieties of welfare states enhance the varieties of citizen professionals that contribute in different ways to contemporary demands on social inclusion and citizenship, and the making of an integrated health workforce (Saks and Kuhlmann, 2006: forthcoming). In particular, the question must be addressed as to whether a strong stakeholder position of the medical profession in Germany and lack of a comprehensive coordination of services provided by other health occupations actually allows for the broadening of the range of providers of care and the epistemological basis of that care. Does this form of regulation produce patterns of "uncertain and evolving dynamic" (Tovey and Adams, 2001, p 695), similar to those described in multidisciplinary models of primary care in the Anglo-American systems? Does it produce a workforce revolution in health care (Davies, 2003)? And what, then, are the 'drivers' for change and the 'enablers' of modernisation in the German system?

An approach on professions as mediators in health care systems provides the opportunity to assess dynamics across different professional groups and macro, meso and micro-levels of change, and to link structure to culture and action dimensions of change. This approach moves beyond the typologies of welfare states and health care systems, and the controversies of marketisation/bureaucratic regulation, and submergence/convergence of health systems. It directs attention towards actors and agency, and the interplay of institutional regulation, cultural norms and formal and informal procedures. Linking change in the professions to changing patterns of governance stimulates a debate on 'professions and the state' (Johnson et al, 1995) and 'professions and the public interest' (Saks, 1995) in a context of changing health policies and user demands. It may also contribute to new approaches in social policy that call for "rethinking governance as social and cultural, as well as institutional practices" (Newman, 2005b, p 197).

Remaking governance, transforming professionalism

New health policies and transformations in society enhance the "fall of an autonomous professional" (Kuhlmann, 2004, p 69) and create a new type of 'citizen professional' and 'citizen consumer'. The emerging new tensions and dynamics caused by the diversity of interests and demands between and within the various groups of providers and stakeholders give rise to a new professionalism in 21st-century societies. This new pattern is markedly different from that of industrialised societies in the late 19th and 20th centuries and the 'golden age' of professions in the postwar period. This perspective brings into view both the transformability of professionalism and the role of the state in targeting and shaping transformations of professionalism.

Modernisation processes in health care touch on a classical issue in sociology, namely the role of the state and bureaucracy, a role that has been the subject of controversy since the work of Marx and Weber. These controversies recur in the study of professions; concepts of the state have been critically reviewed and complemented from different theoretical perspectives (Johnson, 1972; Larson, 1977; Coburn, 1993; Johnson et al, 1995; Macdonald, 1995; Saks, 2003a; Evetts, 2006a). Freidson (2001), among others, claims, for instance, that professionalism stands as a 'third logic' next to market and bureaucracy. However, state regulation itself is undergoing change, and the Weberian definition of the state as an institution that claims a monopoly of legitimate authority and power needs to be reassessed. For example, 'open coordination' makes up a core strategy of the European Union to improve the participation of its various member states (Commission of the European Countries, 2004). New forms of open coordination and network structures are signs of an ongoing development towards the "re-shaping of the state from above, from within, from below" (Reich, 2002, p 1669).

The sociology of the professions offers a framework to further outline these processes of 'reshaping' the state and to assess the enhanced dynamics in health care. By focusing on the professions and professionalism, traditional lines of sociology are taken up and set in a new context. The work of Durkheim (1992 [1950]) and Parsons (1949), for example, highlights the prominent role of the professions in social developments from different theoretical perspectives. From a historical point of view the rise of professionalism and the emergence of professional projects are characteristic of civic societies (Bertilsson, 1990; Burrage and Thorstendahl, 1990; Larson, 1977). Perkin (1989) goes even further and describes the relation between professions and society as the 'rise of professional society'.

Professions continue to play a pivotal role in the concepts of welfare states and the transformation to service-driven societies, which are characterised, on the whole, by an expansion of expert knowledge and professionalism. Moran argues that "the welfare state was a professional state; it depended on professionals both for the expertise needed to formulate policy and to deliver that policy" (2004, p 31). This statement underscores the interdependence of professions, the state and the public, and the need to balance different interests. Against the backdrop of an increasing need to define criteria for the distribution of scarce resources, and to legitimise these decisions in the light of social equality and citizenship rights, professions and professionalism are needed, perhaps more than ever.

Following these argumentations, professions are the 'cornerstones' of welfare states and service societies; and subsequently, with the shifts in the arrangements of welfare states (Hall and Soskice, 2001), and new demands on health care, the professions are also undergoing significant changes. As described elsewhere, "exclusion processes and hierarchies within and between the professions have not been overcome. However, their effectiveness is waning, [...] and new forms of professionalism and 'being a professional' are beginning to emerge" (Blättel-Mink and Kuhlmann, 2003, pp 14-15).

Transformations of professionalism intersect in complex ways with shifts in gender arrangements. A classic pattern of professionalism based on exclusion and hierarchy is closely linked to a gender order that places men and masculinities in the first line; it is related to a 'sexual division' of labour in health care (Parry and Parry, 1976; Witz, 1992). This division is increasingly challenged, for instance, by new professional projects of the predominantly female health occupations and a growing number of women in the medical profession. Gender is therefore an essential dimension when it comes to better understanding the change and persistence of power relations in health care (Davies, 1996; Riska, 2001a; Bendelow et al, 2002; Bourgeault, 2005).

Changes in health care are driven by various forces, which cannot be assessed by simply looking at health policy and institutional regulation. Next to economic constraints, major challenges facing today's health care systems lie, firstly, in a new balance between professional independence and public control, secondly, between the interests and social rights of participation of the various groups of actors in health care, and thirdly, between the individual responsibility of the user and that of the welfare state towards its citizens. With respect to health policy this approach towards professions helps both to bring a broader spectrum of drivers and players into view that may enable change, and to better understand the barriers towards integration and policies introduced from the top down.

Towards context-sensitive approaches: professions, the state and the public as a dynamic triangle

New forms of provider organisation, new actors – like the service users and the various health professions – and new regulatory patterns generate numerous shifts in the health care systems. For example, hierarchies within the medical profession change when general care is assigned a higher value than specialised care. Integrative models of care promote the professionalisation of health professions and occupations; these developments are closely linked to changing gender arrangements. The implementation of market forces and managerialism are further strategies that change the occupational structure and professional identities of the medical profession and incite changes within the 'system of professions' (Abbott, 1988). These developments lead to a situation where the medical profession's calls for autonomy are confronted with the participatory rights of other health care workers and the self-determination of the service users. Changes in work arrangements are called for in this situation, as well as new strategies of legitimising expert knowledge and new forms of building trust in providers.

It must therefore be expected that the restructuring of welfare states, epitomised currently by health care systems, will bring forth new forms of professionalism, new strategies of professionalisation, and new professional projects. Such developments cannot be grasped in terms of 'deprofessionalisation' or 'countervailing powers' (Mechanic, 1991; Light, 1995). Instead of clear effects, what we can expect to see emerging are new tensions that provoke ongoing dynamics and new uncertainties in the health system. Evidence from different health care systems of the *fluidity* of professional boundaries (Saks, 2003b), the *flexibility* of professionalism and professional identities (Hellberg et al, 1999) and *hybrid* forms of organisation and the *context-dependency* of regulation (Dent, 2003; Burau et al, 2004) underscore the need for both new theoretical approaches and comprehensive empirical analysis in order to understand the dynamics and new dimensions of change.

One challenge to research is to disentangle global models and national conditions, discourse and structural change, and the wide range of interests of the players involved in health care systems. Modernisation of health care systems does not simply work as a cascade of regulatory incentives introduced from the top down and leading to frontline changes in the provision of care. As Clarke and colleagues (2005) argue, a conventional dualistic 'from-to' approach – from professionalism to managerialism, from modernity to postmodernity, from self-regulation to new governance and so on – is not convincing. My contention is that a search for the tensions and dynamics 'in-between' these categories is a more promising approach.

Pursuing analysis across disciplines and pulling together different theoretical approaches and research on the professions, health care and social policy may further this search for a more dynamic approach. The demands call for a method that leaves the trodden paths of linear causal logic and instead explores specific 'patterns' (Abbott, 2001) or 'maps' (Burau, 2005) of change. In the present investigation I choose an approach that identifies the 'drivers' and 'enablers' and the 'switchboards' of change in health care and then proceed to examine the dynamics involved empirically (triangulation of methods; see the Appendix). The design is based on four analytical steps and key contentions (see Figure i.1).

The first step is to set out a theoretical framework that places change in health care in the context of modernisation processes in society and links the three arenas of change – state, professions and public. The focus is on professions as mediators and change in this area ('citizen professionals') in relation to new governance ('state') and changing modes of citizenship ('citizen consumers'). The aim is to show that the transition from classical patterns of either state, market or corporatist regulation to more flexible forms of new governance not only impact on the professions in one direction, but also change the actual triangle of professions, the state and citizens in complex and uneven ways.

The second step of analysis focuses, for the main part, on the linkage between professions and the state, and maps out change on macro and meso-levels of regulation; according to an understanding of governance as a complex pattern of regulation, different dimensions are taken into account ('policy, structure, culture'). Set against the backdrop of globalisation and European unification the boundaries between national patterns of welfare state arrangements are increasingly fluid. Accordingly, 'context' cannot be defined merely in nation-specific ways. Analysis of changes in one state needs to be placed in the context of European health systems and global strategies of restructuring of health care, on the one hand, and national transformations and pathways, on the other. I start with, first, a rough plan of analysis of changes in health policy

Figure i.1: Research design: reinventing professions, the state and the public

Step I: Placing professions in context of changing states and public

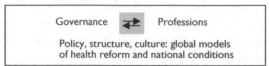

Step II: Mapping change in health care systems

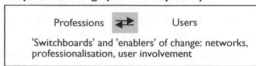

Step III: Assessing dynamics empirically

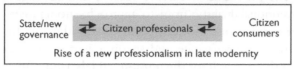

Step IV: Linking dynamics in different arenas of health care

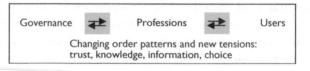

and institutional regulation, organisations and professions, and, especially, quality management as an important element of reform models. These are then made more precise for Germany and set against key concepts of restructuring, namely the establishment of network structures, integrated caring models, quality management and user participation. The focus is on ambulatory care as a key area of restructuring, where the most successful and sustainable changes in the health care system are expected (WHO, 1981; Starfield and Shi, 2002). Methodologically, this part of the work is based on a review of the literature, and additional data sources for Germany, particularly document analysis, statistics and expert interviews with representatives of professional associations and other institutions in health care. I make use of the potential of comparison in a new way: my aim is not to accurately compare various health care systems by means of their differences, but to highlight the travelling of a hegemonic global discourse of 'reform' and 'change' in health care along national highways – and language itself "forms a distinct terrain of political contestation" (Clarke and Newman, 1997, p xiii). This approach directs attention to new tensions and dynamics that move beyond the convergence or submergence of historically embedded patterns of health care systems and shared values. A comparison of global and national patterns of regulation and organisation brings the options and limitations of German corporatism into focus. It helps to identify key arenas – the 'switchboards' and 'enabling actors' – of changes, where dynamics can be assessed empirically.

The third step relates to an in–depth study of these switchboards and enablers, namely the dynamics enhanced through an emerging network culture of the medical profession, changing strategies of professionalisation of the medical profession and health occupations, and user involvement in decision making. Here, the focus is on the linkage between professions and users, and meso and micro-level changes within and between professional groups. Following the structure of the German health system, the medical profession lies at the centre of my investigation. From the wide spectrum of health care workers and professionals I have chosen the physiotherapist and the surgery receptionist, both of whom have very different positions as far as professionalisation, social status and gender relations are concerned. The perspective of the user is brought into the debate by the use of data from members of self-help groups. Different methodological components are taken into account and linked: document analyses and expert information and interviews; a survey of physicians in ambulatory care (n=3,514), based on a written questionnaire; as well as six focus group discussions with the three occupational groups and seven focus groups with the users of health care services. Data were collected, for the main part, from April 2003 to March 2004, in the *Länder* of former West Germany (see the Appendix). My contention is that corporatism is transformed but not replaced; weak state regulation creates new models of medical governance that promote the interests of the medical profession under changing conditions. However, the concepts of professions, professionalism and professionalisation are becoming more diverse and malleable according to new demands.

The fourth step places the empirical results in a broader context of 'changing order patterns' in society, and links dynamics in different arenas of health care systems. Bringing culture into the equation provides the opportunity to combine macro and micro–level findings, and structure and action dimensions of change. This approach moves beyond institutional regulation and brings into view the intersections and tensions within the triangle 'professions, the state and the public'.

Knowledge, information and freedom of choice – the symbolic forces of modernity – 'govern' societies in highly flexible ways, link different actors and interests, build trust in the functioning of societies and reduce social conflict. In these circumstances, classical values and the most powerful tools of professionalism – knowledge, trust and autonomy – are extended to ever more areas of society. At the same time, the knowledge–power knot in professionalism comes under increasing scrutiny. The crucial issue is that cultural patterns of modernity are embedded in new models of 'governing the social' (Newman, 2001) and medical practice (Harrison, 2004; Moran, 2004), and embodied by all players in health care. Accordingly, professions are both the 'objects' of governance and the 'subjects' that govern these practices. Professions and professionalism thus carry a potential for innovation and modernisation of health care, but one that is targeted by state regulation and citizens' demands. This leads back to the relationship between global models and national pathways of change in health care.

Structure of the book

In terms of design, the book follows the four steps of the research design; however, it does not simply move along a linear pathway from one step of analysis to the next. The mediating role of professions between the state and citizens and the rise of new patterns of professionalism provide the connecting link between the chapters. The empirical research findings drawn on for this study thus recur in various chapters. Different analytical levels and perspectives on modernisation processes in health care systems bring into focus the interdependence, ambivalence and contradictions of various areas of institutional changes and shifts in the organising patterns of health care. The book starts with an outline of the theoretical framework and is then divided into three parts: Part I deals with the mapping of change in comparative perspective, Part II with the dynamics of new governance in the German health system and Part III with the rise of a new professionalism in late modernity.

Chapter One links the concept of citizenship as the superstructure of governance of welfare states to research on professions, and sets contemporary changes in historical context. New demands for the accountability of professions and participation of service users mirror shifts in the concept of citizenship towards social inclusion and participation. Professions are expected to exercise both the role of 'officers' and of 'servants' of welfare states (Bertilsson, 1990). Tensions are therefore embedded in professional projects, and health policy attempts to shift the balance towards the 'servant' is changing the tensions. Linking citizenship as a symbol of modernity and professions as contextualised phenomena of welfare states provides a theoretical framework to highlight the transformability of professionalism and to assess the changing relationships between professions, the state and the public in the wake of new demands and modes of governance. This approach helps to overcome a binary logic of 'countervailing powers' between state, market and professions and brings the interdependence and tensions into view.

The first part of the book is related to current changes in health policy and health care systems. Chapter Two provides an overview of developments in different health care systems in order to identify global concepts of modernisation and major areas of change. The US and Britain serve as reference points for market-driven and state-centred systems. In addition, examples from continental Europe and Canada are taken into account. Two key strategies of modernising health care are emerging, namely marketisation and managerialism coupled with consumerism, on the one hand, and the introduction and strengthening of primary care models based on integrated care concepts, on the other. New forms of flexible governance and 'soft bureaucracy' (Flynn, 2004) flank these global patterns of restructuring health care systems. A number of tools that attempt to standardise provider services as well as evidence-based medicine (EBM) give rise to a new pattern of medical governance and 'scientific-bureaucratic medicine', as Harrison (1998) puts it. The common goals of health care systems across countries are integration and coordination of provider services in order to improve both the efficiency and quality of care.

Chapter Three deals with the restructuring in Germany's health system by means of health policy, provider organisation and the occupational structures of physicians, physiotherapists and surgery receptionists. A number of questions are addressed: which changes are implemented from the top down, and how do they translate into frontline changes in the provision of care? What roles do health professions and occupations play in this scenario of change, and which strategies of professionalisation do they advance? The aim of this chapter is to bring reflexivity to the analysis of change, and to highlight the interplay of health policy, organisational change and occupational structure. The findings indicate the coexistence of innovation and conservatism. Corporatism is not replaced but 'modernised' through several elements from new governance. New governance brings the state into corporatist regulation, and at the same, the principle of delegating responsibility to the joint self-administration of stakeholders continues to exist (SVR, 2003, 2005). This stakeholder arrangement is expected to provide the best opportunity to respond to changing demands and reduce social conflict. A state that takes backstage, in turn, enables the medical profession – as the most powerful actor within this arrangement – to successfully fill the vacuum and reassert its power under changing conditions.

Chapter Four links global models and the national context of restructuring in Germany. The aim is to explore nation-specific conditions of modernisation in Germany. The comparative perspective can uncover potential for change, even if it is not yet used in the German context. It reveals that weak drivers for change are increasingly applied to the German health system, while strong drivers are neglected, namely the inclusion of the entire spectrum of health professions and occupations in the regulatory system, and the advancement of a primary care system with multidisciplinary occupational teams. This exploration of strong and weak drivers and enablers of change in Germany provides the basis for a context-sensitive research design of an in-depth empirical study. The switchboards of change are the networks and quality circles of physicians, new professionalisation strategies and the use of professionalism by the health occupations, and the inclusion of the users in the regulatory system; these key arenas of change build the focus of my empirical investigation.

The second part of the book discusses the empirical findings with respect to actor-based changes in the regulation and organising modes of health care systems. Chapter Five outlines how the medical profession takes up the regulatory incentives of managerialism and networking, and how this relates to changes in the corporatist arrangements and the occupational structure. One central finding is that physicians promote the coexistence of new forms of flexible regulation and classical patterns of self-regulation. Furthermore, the rise of a network culture is currently limited to physicians. It does not significantly impact on the organisational structure of ambulatory care and the work arrangements of physicians. In the long run, however, it may impact on the division of labour and the 'institutional environments' in health care as network members expressed more positive attitudes on cooperation with the allied health occupations. Similarly, female physicians' attitudes to patient rights and user participation are more positive than those of male physicians. Consequently, the continuous increase of women in the profession may promote accountability. Taken together, bottom-up changes emanating from the medical profession may further modernisation processes, but in different areas and in various ways, thus provoking different sets of dynamics.

Chapter Six highlights the shifts in professionalism from social exclusion towards more inclusive patterns, which are manifest in new strategies of professionalisation and more contextualised identities. Conservative actors, such as the medical profession, increasingly apply tools from new governance. However, physicians transform the tools aimed at control of providers into successful professionalisation strategies that allow them to avoid tighter control and reassert medical power under changing conditions. The health occupations studied here also make use of the concept of professionalism, but the advantages remain uncertain with respect to occupational control and status. One central issue is a gendered pattern of work and professionalisation, which is transformed but nonetheless alive in new professional projects. The state does not adequately target the potential of professionalism developed from the bottom up to modernise health care systems. This is especially true with respect to the health occupations.

Chapter Seven focuses on the changing role of service users and brings the demands and voices of patients into the equation. Research findings show that the model of 'expert patients' and 'discriminating consumers' is a limited one when applied to health care and the very diverse needs and demands of patients. Generally speaking, patients welcome their new role as informed service users, but at the same time, they sometimes feel incapable of filling this role and seek out doctors' advice in some situations. However, they take the calls for self-responsibility seriously and call for comprehensive information, especially on complementary and alternative therapies. In the German system, with its legally guaranteed choice of providers and a culture of equal access to health care services covered by the Statutory Health Insurance (SHI) funds, health policy's new promises on participation may turn out to challenge the state rather than the professions. New regulatory models may increase the instability of regulation and dissatisfaction of the users.

The third part of the book links the findings to order patterns or 'cultural forces' and leads back to an international debate on restructuring health care and governing the health professions. I choose trust and knowledge as key order patterns of the professions and societies at large; changes in these patterns are closely related to 'information' and 'freedom of choice' as the cultural drivers of modernisation processes (Rose, 1999). These seemingly contradictory developments between seeking trust in medical services and demanding control of providers are the subject of Chapter Eight. I argue that information represents a new technology of building trust on justifiable criteria, which serve as a bridge between different actors in health care, and between experts and lay people. Performance indicators, clinical guidelines and EBM are the 'carriers' of information and the new 'signifiers' of trustworthy relations. A 'disembodied' technology of building trust via information provides new opportunities to improve the social participation of all those labelled 'others'. At the same time, the 'bridge' is controlled by the medical profession, which produces the information that patients, the public and policy makers rely on. Changing strategies and sources of building trust in health care services highlight the interdependency and connectedness of state regulation and the professions.

Chapter Nine puts the knowledge–power knot of professionalism under the spotlight. The power of biomedical knowledge is not simply changed through standardisation and EBM. Moreover, ambivalence is embedded in cognitive standardisation and currently reinforced through economic theory and managerial tools. Both logics claim one single truth and rely on the purported objectivity and neutrality of scientific data. Hereby, the knowledge–power knot of professionalism may even be tightened. At the same time, we can observe a number of fissures, especially those provoked by user demands, that may loosen the knot and shift the balance of power. The cracks are widening where user interests and claims for participation of the various health occupations and alternative therapists coincide and challenge the medical profession from different sides. Once again, the state plays a crucial role when it comes to the inclusion of new actors in the regulatory arrangement and better opportunities to negotiate 'legitimate' knowledge.

The concluding chapter summarises modernisation processes and the dynamics of new governance in health care. It relates back to the reinvention of professions, the state and the public. The focus is on three dimensions of change, namely the rise of a new professionalism; the released tensions and dynamics in the triangle of professions, the state and the public; and the potential, as well as the obstacles, of corporatism and professional self-regulation for modernisation. The options and limitations of a new professionalism, one that is more closely related to social inclusion and participation, are discussed with respect to changing welfare state arrangements and social policy. From this, I conclude by exploring some demands on the future theorising of professions, the state and the public and research into health care and health policy.

ONE

Towards 'citizen professionals': contextualising professions and the state

This chapter stakes out the field for a sociological analysis of changes in health care systems as part of modernisation processes. The concept of citizenship provides the framework to link the issues of regulation and welfare state policy to the study of professions and professionalism. Linking citizenship and professions brings the state back into the study of professions, and in turn, professions into social policy and health care research. This new perspective on the governance of health care moves beyond the controversies between market, state and professional self-regulation. It highlights the role of the professions as mediators between the interests of the body of citizens/state and the individual (research design step I, see Figure i.1). Attention is also directed to the tensions between a global 'superstructure' of governance and the various ways in which states translate this superstructure into practice. I will start with the relationship between professionalism and citizenship and will then come to the current changes, namely consumerism and the calls for integrated care. New approaches in the sociology of professions are discussed; research on complementary and alternative medicine (CAM), as well as midwifery, serve as examples to outline the intersections, tensions and contradictions between state regulation, professional interests and consumer choice. Finally, some preliminary conclusions are drawn as to how to assess current developments in health care in such a way that brings different sets of dynamics into focus, and furthers context-sensitive theoretical approaches.

Citizenship as a superstructure of governance

Citizenship functions as a superstructure of governance. It is both the normative backdrop and a symbol of modernisation processes in Western societies. Dating from the 18th century and continuously developed and transformed under the welfare state system, the concept of citizenship has seen a revival and is currently undergoing yet another transformation within the context of European integration (Bottomore,

1992; Hall and Soskice, 2001; Clarke, 2005). It promises to bridge the contradictions of markets and social equality, of diversity and unification as well as bureaucratic regulation and self-determination.

In health care we can observe the transformations of citizenship 'in action' and assess the promises of social inclusion (Saks and Kuhlmann, 2006: forthcoming). A closer look at this superstructure might provide a promising starting point to gain deeper insights into the underlying order of current developments in health care, its limitations, challenges and options for change. Following Isin and Turner, "negotiations about citizenship take place above and below the state" (2002, p 5). Accordingly, this approach brings new opportunities to overcome the dominant controversy between state-centred/bureaucratic and market-driven strategies of modernising health care.

Most striking for my argument is the role of professions in the concept of citizenship and modernity. Parsons (1949, p 43) described this role as "unique in history" and responsible for any comparable degree of development in major civilisations, and Weber (1978) related the rationalisation of the social order to the rise of the legal profession. Thus, the professions themselves are a signifier of modernity and the main 'translators' of the concept of citizenship into the practice of welfare state services.

The notion of citizenship historically fostered the 'rise of professionalism' (Larson, 1977); numerous new professional projects are being created in the process of expanding social services. Bertilsson (1990) argues that an approach based on professions as the mediators between the state and citizens and a correlation with the power of citizenry "allows us to take a different view on professional power and its accountability: to whom are the professionals accountable, whose interests do they represent?" (1990, p 128). She argues that one can "work out the negotiable status of our social citizenship by means of an interest theory of the professions" (1990, p 131), and directs attention to changes in the power relation between professionals and clients. Following her argument, the current moves towards accountability are likely to transform the status quo of asymmetry and unquestioned trust in medical services. The crucial point is that "individuals as clients or as citizens are allowed to question the basis of expert power and seek to distinguish whether it is based on justificatory reasons or not" (1990, p 130).

This new position of citizens is based on redefinitions of citizenship. In late modernity, individual agency, the construction of self-identity and choice are foremost with regard to citizenship rights (Higgs, 1998; Newman, 2005a). This, in turn, leads to the paradoxical situation that while expert knowledge systems are expanding in the light of increasing 'risks' in society (Beck, 1986) – or 'manufactured uncertainty' as Giddens (1991) calls it – at the same time they are more critically monitored by the public and subject to increasing bureaucratic control. These seemingly paradoxical developments direct attention to changes on different levels and in various areas: both social citizenship and welfare state professionalism date back to the beginning of the 20th century and the emergence of particular types of welfare states. Both concepts are undergoing fundamental transformations, and the welfare state system is itself in transition. Accordingly, change cannot be assessed in a linear sequence of modernisation but must be considered as complex dynamics that may be uneven and contradictory (Clarke, 2004; Newman, 2005b).

The dynamics of social citizenship and the remaking of governance are most visible in health care. This means that precisely those changes, which Bertilsson (1990) addresses – the shifts from unquestioned trust to justifiable reasons – can be assessed empirically. They are made manifest by the calls for transparency, public safety and evidence-based decision making, guidelines for practice and scientific-bureaucratic measurements of care (Harrison, 1998). In addition, the "desire to create consensus" (Higgs, 1998, p 191) and the need for moral criteria for social integration – already emphasised by Durkheim (1992 [1950]) – are most important in health care in order to maintain the legitimacy of social policy and the state. Although restructuring is driven by economics, values are key dimensions of health systems (Light, 1997, 2001). Thus, this arena provides an excellent basis on which to amalgamate citizenship, as a motor of the modernisation of welfare state arrangements, and professionalism, as the regulatory order of health care systems.

Theorising citizenship and professionalism: searching for the connections

The studies of citizenship and those of professions are mainly developed in different scientific discourses with different theoretical references. While citizenship is an issue properly at home in political science, philosophy and welfare state theories, professionalism is more commonly related to the sociology of work and occupation. However, if we look beyond this superficial division, multiple connections and tensions appear. Studying citizenship requires the analysis of welfare state services – which are provided by professionals – and social institutions, such as the educational, health care and law systems. Vice versa, studying the professions calls for a careful analysis of state regulation, markets, cultural and ethical norms, social institutions and power relations. These issues have already been addressed in early work on the professions (Durkheim, 1992 [1950]; Johnson, 1972; Larson, 1977).

More recently the framework of the studies of professions has indeed expanded, especially with respect to regulation and social order. A growing body of literature on regulation in health care highlights current changes (Light, 2001; Allsop and Saks, 2002a; Blank and Burau, 2004). This work opens up perspectives on broader societal developments, such as modernisation, globalisation, neoliberalism and individualisation.

My intention is to further extend the perspectives on regulating the professions to social policy approaches on 'remaking governance' (Newman, 2005a). To understand the changes and challenges of modern societies, it is necessary to understand the role of professions and professionalism (Evetts, 1999). This argument can also be turned on its head: to understand changes in the occupational area of professions, it is necessary to understand its connections to societal change. In this respect, bringing together the various approaches on citizenship and the professions might help to clarify the issues raised in this study (Kuhlmann, 2006a: forthcoming).

Sociological perspectives on citizenship

Theorising citizenship from a sociological perspective can be traced back to early sociologists, such as Weber, Parsons and Durkheim. It was developed further and made an explicit issue by the work of Marshall on "citizenship and social class" (1992 [1950]). The relationship between market forces and social equality, and the power of citizenship as a social order to alter the pattern of social inequality, build the core of Marshall's work: "there is a kind of basic human equality, associated with full community membership, which is not inconsistent with a superstructure of economic inequality" (1992 [1950], p 45). He offers a theoretical framework for combining economic efficiency with social justice. This issue is vital today in the theorising of welfare states and governance (Esping-Andersen, 1996). Numerous authors took up, criticised and expanded the scope of Marshall's ideas. Recent work in particular criticises the ethnocentric and gender bias in the Marshallian legacy and the static view of an evolutionary feature of modern society and citizenship (Siim, 2000). Women do not fit into the framework of citizenship as defined by

Marshall and his followers. This problem goes beyond the exclusion of women and raises the question of how the very different patterns of citizenship and the ambivalence of exclusion and inclusion can be adequately dealt with.

To overcome the problems of a Marshallian model of citizenship Turner introduced a definition of citizenship as a "dynamic social construction" and a "set of practices (juridical, political, economic and cultural), which define a person as a competent member of society, and which as a consequence shape the flow of resources to persons and social groups" (1993, p 2). The author argues for "many diverse and different formulations of the citizenship principle in different social and cultural traditions" (1993, p 9). Turner's work brings ambivalence as an essential feature of citizenship to the fore. Leca argues that citizenship establishes a double relation in terms of interests:

> Those individuals who consider their interests as properly served through citizenship are recognised as the best citizens, and those who possess the most 'capital' (material, cultural or technological) are recognised as the most competent. On the other hand, citizenship is also a resource which permits more of the socially disempowered to acquire a greater political competence and to defend their interests more effectively. (1992, p 30)

In Leca's sense, the idea of citizenship is currently incorporated into the debates on consumerism and stakeholder regulation. This is empirically visible in 'third way' approaches and theorised by Giddens (1998) as 'renewal of social democracy'. Research into health care confirms and further outlines the connections: "The Third Way approaches emphasise user empowerment, democratic renewal, social inclusion, stakeholding, and communitarian notions of active citizenship" (Baggott, 2002, p 42). Despite the many calls for participation, however, the main question of the theories of citizenship – already addressed by Turner (1993; Isin and Turner, 2002) – remains largely unsolved. What exactly are the regulatory mechanisms that advance or hinder inclusion and social participation as major trends in Western nation states? To get closer to these issues it might be fruitful to go beyond the scope of theories of citizenship and to take a look at the studies of professions.

The professional: a blueprint for the 'ideal citizen'

Marshall already laid out the pathways for relating professions and citizenship. With respect to the 'social element' of citizenship in the 19th century he points out the significance of the educational system and social services as "the institutions most closely connected with it" (Marshall, 1992 [1950], p 8). These institutions are precisely the traditional arenas of professionalised work and professional organisations. The links between citizenship and professionalism continue on the level of actors. With regard to the Hungarian concept of citizenship, Turner writes: "the idea of the educated civil servant as the leading example of the citizenship was a common development" (1993, p 11). Similarly, in the German tradition the "*Bürgertum* was a product of the city who, through training and education, achieved a civilized mastery of emotions; the result was a new status group, the *Bildungsbürgertum*" (Turner, 1992, p 50). It is exactly this *Bildungsbürger*, identified by Turner as the product of citizenship, that marks the beginning of an emerging professionalism in Germany, and the term is sometimes used synonymously with the Anglo-American 'professional' (Burrage and Thorstendahl, 1990).

Within a republican doctrine of citizenship the approach of this civil servant or *Bürger* is that of "a free and independent person", but at the same time an "officer of the community, whose personal qualities and attributes are therefore a matter of legitimate concern for the community as a whole" (Hindress, 1993, p 21). The notion of autonomy is central to the different concepts of citizenship, whether republican, liberal or social democratic (Siim, 2000), but most strongly advocated in liberalism. The descriptions of ideal citizens highlight the similarities of the citizenship role and the status of professionals as portrayed in ideal-typical classifications. The 'autonomous' professional is expected to act according to the ethics of 'professional altruism' as regulatory powers against the values of the market place (Freidson, 2001). The professional thus seems to fit best the picture of an ideal citizen and the goals of social citizenship developed in classical theory of citizenship.

These connections direct our attention to the regulatory dimensions of professionalism. Following Offe, "becoming a 'good' citizen is a demanding project, both for the individuals themselves and for all those professions [...] involved in the formation of the qualities of citizens" (2003, p 297). The author argues that this formation of a citizen requires a reference unit that is adopted by individual agents as guiding their political judgements. Within this reference unit the "appropriate decision criterion, or mix of criteria" and "knowledge" are important components of the citizenship role (Offe, 2003, p 298). The significance of legitimate criteria for decision making actually increases with the emerging 'project of the self' (Higgs, 1998) and the transformation of state authority.

If we apply this more general statement on knowledge and a widely accepted value system to the field of health care, the links to professionalism become obvious. Trust in the qualification and competence of the medical profession and in the biomedical knowledge and science system provide the required reference unit for the political institutions, the occupations, patients and the public. Professionalism is a resource for legitimating welfare state policy, and serves to iron out the contradictions between regulation and individualisation (Harrison and Ahmad, 2000).

These briefly sketched examples are proof of the relationship between professionalism and citizenship on the level of structure, culture and actors, especially in health care. As normative concepts, both draw on an 'autonomous' individual, and both are regulatory mechanisms working 'at a distance' (Miller and Rose, 1990) to govern social institutions, as well as individual practices. Turner has recently argued that "we can think about citizenship as providing legal solutions for the management of individuals and populations" (2004, p 268). A further striking similarity of both concepts is the underlying structure of hegemonic masculinity, which denies women – and all those labelled as 'others' – full access to citizenship and to the professions, too. And thirdly, as far as social structure and action are concerned, professionals are represented in the institutions of the welfare states and directly involved in policy processes. In a knowledge-based and service-oriented society, professionalism and the standardisation of knowledge are becoming increasingly significant, and health care is a particularly decisive arena of change.

Citizenship and the rise of professionalism

Historically, the concepts of social citizenship and professionalism are amalgamated in a way that enhances professional projects and strengthens the regulatory power of professionalism. These developments have been elegantly described by Larson (1977) as the "rise of professionalism" in terms of market power and social closure within the matrix of capitalism. In Larson's model, professionalisation is "an attempt to translate one order of scarce resources – special knowledge and skills – into another – social and economic rewards" (Larson, 1977, p xvii). These processes require an internal unification of the professions, which is achieved by "conflict and struggle around who shall be included or excluded" (Larson, 1977, p xii). Further conditions are actual or potential markets for the skilled services of labour (Larson, 1979).

Next to markets the state was the key actor in the emergence of professional projects. In his early work Johnson discusses the relationship between the state and the professions in terms of power and control, and directs attention to the impact of welfare state policies:

> Considerations of social welfare, social and preventative medicine, law reform, etc, will bring practitioners more explicitly into the political arena. The 'authoritative' pronouncement common under the system of professionalism gives way to the incorporation of practitioners, as advisers and experts, within the context of government decision-making. (1972, p 84)

Johnson, states, "an industrialising society is a professionalising society" (1972, p 9), and Moran (2004) continues this statement with a definition of the welfare state as a professional state. The developing welfare states had a vital interest in the expansion of professional projects. As they promised access to social services for citizens, they had to provide and expand the markets for professionalised work. From the perspective of the public, these services offered by the professions beCAMe a gauge for the success of the aims of welfare states to translate the concept of social citizenship into the practice of social services. From the perspective of the professions, the growing significance of knowledge and state regulation and the protection of qualification opened up new chances for participation by transforming knowledge into economic benefits; knowledge is the 'currency' of capitalist societies (Larson, 1977) and competition in the occupational field (Abbott, 1988). These processes provoked changes in the class structure of societies, and enabled the professionals to struggle for upward social mobility and to qualify for the epithet of 'ideal citizen'.

As outlined by Larson, professionalism also serves as an ideological model for "justifying inequality of status and closure of access in the occupational order" (1977, p xviii). The state made use of professionalism, both as a strategy for participation in the 'merits' of civic society and as a strategy to legitimise exclusion. In this latter sense, the regulatory mechanisms of professionalism and professional self-regulation can serve to reduce social conflicts. Self-regulation is assumed "to produce higher levels of trust between the regulated and the regulatory bodies than is the case with direct regulation" (Baggott, 2002, p 34; see Stacey, 1992). Ambivalence and flexibility of the superstructure of citizenship are therefore also a component of professionalism that allows for various transformations and provokes ongoing dynamics.

More recent work emphasises the different roads of professionalisation, its diversity and the differences between the actors who are able or unable to make use of professionalism in the most effective way. The growing call for diversity raised by theories of governance and citizenship (Clarke and Newman, 1997) is parallelled by the research on professions. Comparative studies reveal the differences between nations and between occupational groups (Dent, 2003; Saks, 2003b; Svensson and Evetts, 2003a). In the same vein as in the debates on welfare states and citizenship, the introduction of gender highlights some of the shortcomings of classical approaches and typologies. Feminist research provides convincing examples of the differences within professional groups and the ongoing development leading from exclusionary strategies to the tactics of inclusion (Riska, 2001a; Kuhlmann, 2003). There is a rather uniform tendency in different welfare states, which points to the rise of a *new* professionalism, which is different from that of industrial society of earlier times. I will come back to this issue in detail in the second and third parts of the book. At this juncture, I wish to set out the lines of new challenges on theory and research into governing health care.

New approaches on the professions

In line with the growing service sector, professionalism has expanded from the classical professions to new occupational fields and groups, and is used by new actors (Evetts, 2003). The health care system provides numerous examples for new professional projects of formerly subordinated occupations, such as nursing and midwifery (Davies, 2002a; Bourgeault et al, 2004; Dahle, 2006: forthcoming), or new groups of alternative and complementary therapists (Kelner et al, 2003; Saks, 2003b). This sector also demonstrates how professionalism is utilised and transformed by new actors from outside the system of health professions, especially by means of management and changing health policies (Davies, 2003; Kirkpatrick et al, 2005). Professionalism offers new opportunities for managing diversity and, in this sense, represents the 'reference unit' of decision making that bridges different actors and interests.

Against the backdrop of diversity there is an increasing need for a 'reference unit', outlined as an important condition of social citizenship (Offe, 2003). In late modernity there is no such ethical reference unit within societies that can lay claim to being an overall legitimacy for decision making. This ethical gap can be appropriately filled by professional knowledge and formalised expert knowledge systems, which provide seemingly objective and neutral data and criteria for decision making. 'Trust in numbers' (Porter, 1995) and evidence-based medicine are widely accepted by the public, politics, experts and laypeople alike. Such results count as the 'gold standard' of health care, against which all decision making is to be measured (Timmermans and Berg, 2003). In this sense, the orthodox medical knowledge system is the most powerful regulatory mechanism, and physicians the most trusted group in society, although changes are underway in both areas (Calnan and Sanford, 2004; Kuhlmann, 2006b). Within the scope of governance of changing welfare states the professionals and professionalism are needed to legitimise political decisions and to maintain trust in social services, especially in view of leaner budgets and more demanding customers.

The increasing significance of professionalism is echoed by recent shifts in theory and research on professions that direct attention to professionalism as social order. This research takes up a classical theme of the sociology of professions (for example, Parsons, 1949; Durkheim, 1992 [1950]) and reformulates it. Since the 1990s, professionalism has been increasingly linked to the work of Foucault. This approach bridges regulation on different levels; state and institutional regulation and individual action are all related to discourse and a changing technology of regulating societies called 'governmentality' (Foucault, 1979; Dean, 1999). Fournier describes professionalism as the "new software" (1999, p 291), which allows for the control of flexible forms of organisations, paid work and "more fundamentally, employees' subjectivities" (1999, p 293). She also points out that this control is never total, but opens up "new possibilities for resistance and subversion as the meaning of professionalism gets contested" (1999, p 302). Evetts (2003, 2006a) further highlights the flexibility and the 'double standard' of professionalism as an effective instrument of occupational change and control. Again, the interrelations with the concept of citizenship lie ahead. Both concepts can be used to enhance and defend status and power but also to empower those at the margins.

A Foucauldian approach may be exciting but it is not fully convincing. The challenge is to 'materialise' discourse and distinguish the various ways it is used and the social conditions that determine the translation of discourse into practice. Evetts, by taking on

McClelland's (1990) suggestion, stresses a distinction between "professionalism from above" and "professionalism from within" (2003, p 26). She argues for the necessity to assess the very different realities and social effects of these forms. The medical profession clearly provides an example of 'professionalism from within' because it has the power to set the agenda for health policy and the whole range of health care services. However, this agenda is not necessarily in line with conservative forces. Clarke and Newman (1997), arguing from a social policy approach, direct attention to an innovative potential of professionalism:

> Welfare professionalism was at least partially open to the attempts by the new social movements to socialise definitions of social problems, and become one of the sites in which issues about 'discrimination', 'empowerment' and inequalities of different kinds were played out. (1997, p 11)

Professions may serve as a conservative force in health care and at the same time, further social inclusion and participation in a particular context. Consequently, there is a need to assess the tensions between conservatism and innovation. Burau recently introduced a theoretical framework of "actor-based governance" that offers a more systematic analysis of context and the interplay between context and actors (2005, p 114). Regarding the legal profession and the challenges of European integration, Olgiati argues for a "Janus-headed approach" in order to fully grasp "contingency and discontingency, alteration and manifestation between facts and values, actions and wills, practical instruments and their cultural significations, eg discourses" (2003, p 73).

These briefly sketched perspectives on the professions highlight regulatory mechanisms that go beyond institutional regulation and occupational structure. They direct attention to actors and cultural rules, and point to the 'blind spots' of a Foucauldian approach, which amalgamates different social positions and interests of actors to one pattern of order. In the following sections I will argue the need for further theoretical and empirical investigation to better understand the tensions between professions, the state and the public and the dynamics of new governance. The challenges of integrative care concepts and consumerism serve as examples to underscore my argument.

Integration and cooperation: changing demands on the professions

The making of an integrated health workforce and consumer involvement in the health policy process are clearly related to changing modes of citizenship and are shaped by these ideas. To access the impact on health professions, Evetts' (2003) suggestion may be helpful to distinguish between the classical professions and those that were formerly excluded and governed 'from above'. Here, I would like to add a third dimension of professionalism – one that goes beyond occupational control – namely the 'use' of professionalism by the service users. This latter group refers to professionalism, especially when it comes to public and individual judgements on the quality of service and the resources needed to fund it. Users act as transformers of professionalism 'from the outside'. They provoke changes in the medical profession and the system of occupational groups, and also in the epistemological foundation of professional knowledge and its methods of testing and evaluation. Consequently, a dichotomous concept of professionalism from within or from above does not fully grasp the interconnected social changes that govern the health professions.

The studies of professionalisation of CAM provide convincing examples for the complex and flexible relationships between user demands, integrative care and occupational change (Saks, 2003b; Kelner et al, 2004). They also highlight the tensions between culture and discourse, on the one hand, and regulation and action that are based on professional interests, on the other. Saks argues that the professionalisation of CAM providers, such as chiropractors, acupuncturists and osteopaths, is in line with public interest and increasing demand for these services, but cannot be seen as a defensive reaction to the medical challenge in a favourable climate of public opinion:

> It can also bring positive benefits to those involved in terms of the enhanced income, status and power associated with exclusionary closure, as well as the satisfaction of working in a well-regulated profession. That said, groups of CAM therapists have followed a number of different avenues to professionalization. (2003c, p 230)

In drawing on historical analysis and a comparison of Britain and the US, Saks reveals that the success of these strategies varies according to national patterns of regulation. The more rapid move towards integration of alternative medicine in the US compared to Britain, according to Saks, is in part related to cultural differences. Most important, however, are the "differential legal terms on which the exclusionary social closure of medicine was based" (2003b, p 89). To paraphrase the results of this study, a regulatory framework of health care that allows anyone to offer CAM in general seems to work against the inclusion into medical care, even in the face of public demand. Furthermore, the author shows that inclusion of CAM in health care does not necessarily meet the demands on integrative care as long as multidisciplinary teamwork, intersectorial collaboration and bottom-up thinking are not brought into practice (Saks 2003b, p 161). The comparative approach reveals that options for integrated caring concepts and inclusion of new occupational groups are, at least in part, the outcome of specific forms of state regulation.

Additionally, I would like to direct attention to similarities between the inclusion of CAM and gender issues into health care. In the US the integration of women into medical research, especially with respect to the randomised controlled trial (RCT), and the mainstreaming of gender into health care plans and evaluations (Healy, 1991; McKinley et al, 2001) make most progress in comparison with European countries. Within Europe, the advancement of European unification serves as a catalyst of gender equality as a criterion for decision making. However, there are significant differences between the member states, and Germany clearly lacks a systematic inclusion of gender issues, even in the new models of health care (Kuhlmann and Kolip, 2005). Interestingly, the provision of CAM services is excluded from SHI care and provision not limited to a specific professional group. In this respect, Germany shows precisely those regulatory patterns identified as barriers towards more inclusive health care services (Saks, 2003b). Similarities between the inclusion of CAM practitioners and gender issues in different health systems direct attention towards the significance of regulatory frameworks that may either block or further the integration of all those labelled 'others' in the landscape of biomedicine.

Most interestingly for my study, looking at the regulation of the medical profession does not tell the whole story of social inclusion and exclusion in health care. Moreover, the regulation of all those groups on the margins or outside the orthodox medical system provides a key to better understanding the options for a more inclusive professionalism. New perspectives open up if we apply the findings to the German health system. Corporatism and a strong stakeholder position of the medical profession, which are viewed in welfare state research as major barriers to innovation, are only partly responsible for the laggard pace of restructuring in Germany. Moreover, lack of professionalisation of the health occupations and their weak position in the regulation system are equally important barriers. I will come back to this in the following chapters and assess its potential for the modernisation of Germany's health care system against the backdrop of my empirical data.

Consumerism: a new regulatory order in the public service sector

Consumerism is a powerful discourse in health care and an important 'tool' to transform the aims of social citizenship according to changing concepts of welfare state governance and state responsibility for public services. While user involvement is continually gaining ground, its emergence dates back to the 1960s and 1970s. For example, Gartner and Riessman (1978) already pointed out the advantages of 'active consumers' in terms of quality of social care, efficiency of service and empowerment of users. Some elements of consumerism, like empowerment and self-determination, are related to the medical counter-culture emerging from the 1960s onwards. In particular, the women's health movement was the most powerful motor for change, as it challenged the structure and normative ground of paternalist and biomedical-centred health care systems (BWHBC, 1971). Other aspects, such as calls for self-responsibility of patients and the transformation of social relations in health care into the logic of markets and customers, are the outcome of neoliberal developments and managerialism in the 1990s.

Consumerism draws on different and in part contradictory ideological concepts and includes different interests. Clarke and colleagues (2005) highlight these different dimensions of consumerism and its transformations against the backdrop of third way politics in Britain. The authors convincingly argue that the discourse of consumerism provides new options for participation and social inclusion, and at the same time, may provoke new social inequalities and instabilities of regulation.

The appeal of consumerism derives from its ability to connect economic benefits and social participation:

> The enterprising customer-consumer is imagined as an empowered human being – the moral centre of the

enterprising universe. Within the discourse of enterprise customers/consumers are constituted as autonomous, self-regulating and self-actualizing individual actors, seeking to maximize the worth of their experience to themselves through personalized acts of choice in a world of goods and services. (DuGay and Salaman, 1992, p 623)

Consumerism as a discourse marches in step with the construction of an 'autonomous self' and 'reflexive actor' dominant in Western societies (Giddens et al, 1994). Lupton highlights "a congruence between the notion of the 'consumerist' patient and the 'reflexive' actor. Both are understood as actively calculating, assessing and, if necessary, countering expert knowledge and autonomy with the objective of maximizing the value of services such as healthcare" (1997, p 374).

The type of subject portrayed in this consumerist model is non-differentiated (Lupton, 1997; Clarke et al, 2005). Gender, class, 'race' or biographical experiences are not taken into account as determining factors in decision making. However, consumerism favours those individuals who are able or willing to act according to 'rational choice' and market laws. While consumerism fosters inclusion processes, it does so at the expense of certain social groups that are excluded because they are not 'market-savvy'. Freedom of choice – the appealing promise of late modernity – seems first and foremost to be an option for all those who fit the categories of 'normality' rather than the sick, old and poor (Williams, 2003).

These exclusionary tactics produce social inequality, which is legitimised by the 'autonomous' decision making of physicians and 'savvy' patients. This causes a shift in responsibility from the macro-political level of welfare states to the micro-political level of the users. The concept of citizenship in terms of solidarity and welfare is redefined in terms of the right to choose. According to Miller and Rose (1990), the programmes of government are evaluated in terms of the extent to which they enhance choice. Higgs argues that the shift in the concept of citizenship "represents a change in the organising principle of state welfare" rather than a retreat from the welfare state (1998, p 188). Harrison and Mort characterise this shift as a new "technology of legitimation" (1998, p 60), but also acknowledge the actual and possible changes evoked by user involvement.

Consumerism reinforces the need for a normative reference unit. The medical expert knowledge system provides the most accepted normative ground, thereby securing the most efficient use of consumerism in terms of state regulation. Similarly, the role of professionals as mediators between the interests of the state and citizens is strengthened as the government profits from the very high levels of public trust in physicians. Despite its challenges to the medical profession, consumerism does not generally function as a 'countervailing power' to the professions but gives rise to a new pattern of professionalism and opens new fields for its use. The power of professionalism does not shrink, but expands. However, new actors, such as service users, may transform the concept of professionalism itself and the strategies to professionalise, thereby provoking shifts in the power relations in health care.

The key role of the state becomes apparent if consumerism is viewed as a changing pattern of regulation related to new governance. Allsop and colleagues conclude from research in Britain that "health consumer groups are now viewed as legitimate stakeholders", particularly as they bring in resources "that the government finds useful in the present context" (2002, p 62). Allsop's argument points to the fact that states may define and use the concept of consumerism in different ways depending on the actual resources the users of health care are expected to bring in. From this perspective, the current patterns of consumerism in the Anglo-American health systems do not have the ultimate goal of 'putting patients first' and improving citizenship rights; these patterns also serve the interests of governments. A stronger advancement of consumerism in the US and Britain compared to Germany, therefore, is not simply an inevitable outcome of professional self-regulation. Moreover, the differences mirror different patterns of governing health care.

Professions, the state and the users as interdependent players: the case of midwifery

The complexity of conditions of change and the different impact on diverse occupational and social groups of users in terms of professionalisation, equality and quality of care are particularly manifest in research on midwifery. These studies highlight that, apart from consumer choice, state regulation and professional interests – especially the power of the medical profession – are key dimensions in understanding the success of professional projects (Bourgeault et al, 2004). I would like to refer to this work to underscore the intersections and tensions, and related to this, a need for context-sensitive approaches.

The professionalisation of midwifery is currently making progress in a number of health systems. This echoes the call for women-centred care and critique of the medicalisation of childbirth, especially from the realm of the women's health movement. The strategies and social effects, however, vary significantly between states. A comparison with the professionalisation of midwives in the US and Canada shows that stronger state regulation has a positive effect on midwives' professional goals when the interests of the latter coincide with those of the state (Bourgeault and Fynes, 1997). According to the authors, a growing tendency for state support for midwives' demands was apparent in both countries, although efforts to professionalise were more successful in Canada. This is put down to the fact that, in comparison with the US, physicians in Canada have less power, while the state has higher powers of intervention.

Here, I would like to call to mind Witz's (1992) historical research on gender and professionalisation, which confirms the impact of state regulation on the success of female professional projects. Witz compares legalist tactics and 'credentialism' related to the attempts to gain support from within the professions. She is able to demonstrate that credentialist strategies are more homogeneous and thus favour exclusionary strategies, whereas the heterogeneous character of legalistic strategies opens 'windows of opportunity'. The results show that legalistic tactics have a more positive impact on women's chances in the medical profession and female professional projects than credentialist ones. This relationship is also confirmed with respect to the entrance of women in the medical and dental profession in Germany (Kuhlmann, 2001, 2003).

The challenge of today is to add to the pattern of state regulation the forces of increasing marketisation and consumerism. Users are most effective in provoking changes to cut costs and maintain "legitimacy vis-à-vis a female electorate" (Bourgeault and Fynes 1997, p 1061) when their interests are in line with the aims of the state. A comparison of the situation of Canadian, British, German and US midwives also underlines the ambivalence of state intervention, professionalisation and working conditions: the professional status of midwives is rising in all countries. It is reported, however, that the rise in status is coupled with higher stress levels and burn-out syndrome, because of users' calls for permanent availability, which increases working hours (Sandall et al, 2001, p 134). The authors emphasise that the collective rise in status of this group does not necessarily lead to better working conditions and that results vary from individual to individual. Consequently, occupational interests of midwives to improve their status within the system of health care do not necessarily coincide with women's interest in high-quality and self-determined care. A comparative study of developments in obstetrics in Britain, Finland

and Canada reveals that while state regulation can further the professionalisation of midwifery, it does not necessarily improve the quality of care; for example, changes may actually increase the fragmentation of care (Wrede et al, 2001).

Research on midwifery shows that specific chances of professionalisation cannot be grasped by simply looking at levels of regulation – whether state or market/consumer choice – but by analysing the interactions of various players and regulatory policies. This is where developments in other social fields and superposed regulatory systems, such as the gendered division of labour and the public–private divide, become relevant (Benoit, 1999). Research on midwifery also highlights that quality of care can neither be reduced to professsionalisation nor to consumer choice and satisfaction; it needs additional criteria and assessment, especially with respect to the organisation of care. The aims to improve equity of care, workers' rights and consumer choice do not fit as easily as concepts of restructuring of health care promise (Benoit, 1999). Taken together, the results call for new approaches that can grasp the interplay of different regulatory mechanisms and diverse actors with sometimes contradictory interests (Bourgeault, 2005).

Professions and citizenship: some preliminary conclusions

The linking of theories of citizenship and governance to theoretical concepts from the sociology of professions helps to assess the changes in health care in a broader framework of processes of modernisation. This chapter has shown that the historical ties and tensions between professions and social citizenship are continuously transformed. The rise of a new professionalism in late modernity is different from the classical patterns hitherto observed in the industrialised societies. Consequently, the tensions are also changing and new, not fully predictable, dynamics are emerging. I will come back to these issues in the third part of the book. For the moment, I would like to direct attention towards the ambivalence embedded in the model of citizenship as a resource for both legitimising and balancing social inequality, and claiming participation and equality.

Ambivalence is transferred to the professions. Bertilsson calls this the "duality of the modern professional practice finding itself torn between the body–citizen (the state) and the individual person" (1990, p 131). She makes the point that it "is not easy to be an executor of legitimate power and at the same time serve those who are the subjects of that same power" (1990, p 131). Thus, tensions and conflicts of interests are deeply embedded in the demands on professions, and release ongoing dynamics into the health care system and the health workforce. These tensions cannot simply be overcome by individual actors, whether professionals or service users. They can, however, be either reduced or reinforced by different models of state regulation, as research into CAM and midwifery shows.

Regarding theory and research, further investigation is needed to link the study of professions to the debates on remaking governance, and the changing role of governments and 'people' (Clarke, 2004; Newman, 2005a). For the main part, theorising the state from the perspective of professions has been left to Marxist perspectives, which were especially dominant in the 1970s (for instance, Johnson, 1972), as well as to neo-Weberian and, more recently, to Foucauldian approaches. A growing body of literature from welfare state and social policy research, however, throws up new perspectives that have not yet been fully reviewed with respect to professions. Linking this research to the study of professions might contribute to fresh insights on current developments in health care (Moran, 1999; Burau, 2005). A systematic connection may also strengthen the ties between sociology and social policy, and, by doing so, continue the tradition of approaches that place research in the area of professions in a broader framework of social theories, such as those of Marx, Weber and Durkheim. Today's challenges, however, are to overcome the limitations that these 'grand narratives' impose, and to explore new connections that are more sensitive to context, gender and diversity.

The present work responds to the need for a critical review of theoretical approaches in putting emphasis on context and empirically assessing different trajectories of change, different groups of stakeholders and players in health care, and different 'sets of dynamics'. Context is defined, firstly, with respect to the interconnectedness of professions, the state and the public, and secondly, the interplay of global models and national conditions of restructuring health care (see the Introduction to this volume). I do not claim that with this approach we can be sure to escape the 'iron cage of binary thinking' embedded in Western societies and modernity; in particular, the debate on convergence and submergence of national health systems, and the assumption that change in health care shows up in linear sequence, like consumerism, managerialism, marketisation, and so on. I do hope, however, that it will contribute to comprehensive empirical data in order to make 'informed decisions' on the dynamics of new governance in health care and its potential to serve the needs and demands of changing societies.

Part I
Mapping change in comparative perspective

The first part of this book deals with the translation of modernisation processes and changing patterns of citizenship into the politics and practice of health care. What are the drivers and key strategies of modernisation? What key areas and 'switchboards' of social change can we identify? What role do changing regulatory frameworks play? What dynamics are released by these processes, and how can the latter be determined empirically with respect to Germany? These are the questions addressed in the following three chapters. Restructuring of health care is an international phenomenon. However, the uniform rhetoric of global debates on reform clashes head on with the diversity of welfare states. The aim of Part I is to map the changes on levels of policy, structure and culture to better understand the dynamics of global models and national restructuring (research design step II, see Figure i.1). Changes in institutional regulation and health policy, in the organisation of care and within the professions serve as rough categories to draw a more comprehensive map of modernisation processes and the dynamics involved. In addition, the various forms of management and control of providers are taken into account, where new patterns of medical governance are manifest in frontline changes.

Part 1
Mapping change in comparative perspective

Global models of restructuring health care: challenges of integration and coordination

Marketisation is the preferred modernisation strategy and an engine driving many changes in health care. It is introduced into very different systems, flanked by concepts of new public management (NPM) and decentralisation. The role of the service user is thereby becoming ever more important. The second line of development is based on the Alma Ata Declaration of the World Health Organization (WHO, 1981), which calls for the establishment of primary care as the solution to health care problems. The introduction of new models of primary care counts as central to the success of reforms. Marketisation and a radical shift away from highly technical in-patient care to primary care cut deeply into the grown structures and norms of Western health systems. New models of integration and a coordination of provider services and expertise – such as that of the allied health professions, alternative therapists and patients – call for both new models of governance and new patterns of professionalism. A network structure of governance and tighter managerial control are assumed to be the most effective ways to improve the quality of care. The challenges, changes and dynamics of these developments are the themes of this chapter.

Hybrid forms of governance

To a high degree, reform concepts in the health sector depend on policy and system reform (WHO, 2000; Hill, 2002), and attempt to strengthen primary care (Donaldson et al, 1996; Light, 2001; Tovey and Adams, 2001). A comparative study of 15 health systems concludes: "The stronger the primary care, the lower the costs. Countries with very weak primary care infrastructures have poorer performance on major aspects of health" (Starfield and Shi, 2002, p 201). Processes of change are connected to the growing weight accorded to the health of the population on political agendas (World Bank, 1993). There is hardly another area where justice and equality enjoy higher relevance than in the area of health care.

The interplay between tighter economic resources and changes in the system of care, as well as globalisation and European unification, call for new forms of regulation. The introduction and expansion of marketisation and managerialism are the favoured answers to new demands. Although the 'simple-minded marketisation' (Reich, 2002) is wishful thinking, developments provoke changes in the regulatory frameworks and the arrangement of players. Furthermore, health care is not simply governed at political and institutional levels, but shaped by cultural order patterns, informal modes of regulation, and change in other social areas. Such overlapping influences are, for instance, changes in gender relations and the changing needs and wishes of users, for example, for CAM therapies. The traditional classification of 'market, state, corporatism' does not take these interdependencies into account; in particular, users are missing from this triad. The following section outlines the connectedness and tensions of different regulatory mechanisms.

Interplay of market, state and corporatism

Health research has developed its own classification of systems that differs from the typology of welfare states developed by Esping-Andersen (1996) and his followers. At the macro-political level, three models of regulation are identified: market, state and corporatist actors (Blank and Burau, 2004). The US represents the prototype of a market-driven system; Britain and other Anglo-Saxon countries stand as examples of state-centred systems, Germany is a classical example of corporatism. Market-driven and corporatist systems fit the welfare state typology of 'liberal' and 'corporatist' systems, at least in part, while the differences of the classification schemes are more obvious in the case of Britain, which is labelled 'liberal' in terms of welfare state theory.

Despite widespread debate on classifying welfare states and health systems (for instance, Moran, 1999; Freeman, 2000), new regulatory policies and the move towards marketisation observed in all health systems enhance dynamics that challenge the typology itself. The impact of neoliberal market policies stretches far beyond changes on the level of market and competition. Although such policies attempt to weaken the role of the state they actually lead to a stronger need for state regulation in order to counter market failure and system abuse (Reich, 2002). New patterns of governance are turning from substantive to more procedural regulation and hybrid incentive structures (Saltman, 2002). Flynn (2004) characterises the new patterns as 'soft bureaucracy' in contrast to classical models of bureaucratic regulation based on hierarchy; and Harrison (1998) introduces the term 'scientific-bureaucratic medicine' that most clearly emphasises an amalgamation of science and bureaucracy.

This hybridisation is not merely a result of changes in certain national health systems. It is also a reaction to the globalisation and increasing diversity of actors. Coburn argues that "globalization provides a major rationale for the introduction of market principles and materially reinforces the role of those agents, corporations or political parties, supporting neo-liberal politics" (1999, p 151). In future, not only must many more actors be taken into account, but also new and potentially changing arrangements between multinational corporations – including non-governmental organisations (NGOs) – and local states. Markets and states do not necessarily stand, therefore, in opposition to one another but function as complementary regulatory instances (Newman, 2001). The issue, therefore, is not one of 'more' or 'less' state or 'more' or 'less' market in health care, but a transformation of the patterns of regulation into a complex system of new governance.

In a similar manner to the market and the state, corporatism and marketisation are often seen as two opposing poles of the regulatory structures. Here, too, the relationship is more complex. In Britain, for instance, evidence exists of a tendency towards stronger corporatist structures arising from market orientation (Allsop, 1999). Corporatist political activity and forms of regulation are also growing in importance with regard to the regulation of drugs in the European Union (EU) and in Britain (Abraham, 1997). Turning our attention to the medical profession as a central corporatist actor, we continue to find contradictory evidence. On the one hand, US authors, especially, proceed on the principle of the existence of 'countervailing powers' (Mechanic, 1991) between diverse forms of regulation and predict a loss of power and autonomy of professions owing to neoliberal developments and managerialism in health care (Light, 1995; Freidson, 2001). On the other hand, a number of studies, especially recent research from Europe, do not support the hypothesis of an overall loss of power of the medical profession or a deprofessionalisation process but direct attention to more complex change (Schepers and Casparie, 1999; Dent, 2003; Blank and Burau, 2004; Gray and Harrison, 2004).

From whichever vantage point we look at the interrelation between market, state and corporatism, it is becoming apparent that change in this relationship does not follow a linear sequence. Moreover, different regulatory patterns are amalgamating and conflicting in ways that classical categories – whether they are taken from welfare state or health system typologies – can no longer grasp. The term 'hybrid' (Saltman, 2002; Dent, 2003) or the concept of 'maps' as used by Blank and Burau (2004; Burau, 2005) are, for the moment, useful constructions to describe hitherto unknown forms of regulation.

From a geographical perspective the hybridisation of regulation is parallelled by the development of an increased decentralisation of health care (Atkinson, 2002; Reich, 2002). The degree of decentralisation is considered an important criterion when it comes to the evaluation of health systems. When set in the context of current developments, however, this classification is also seen to fail. Burau's comparative study of nursing in Britain and Germany demonstrates that "the differences observed seem to turn the existing typologies on their head" (1999, p 251). In the German health system, generally considered to be decentralised, the boundaries between occupational groups seem to be centrally regulated from the 'bottom–up' perspective of the local level, which leads to considerable restrictions in the professionalisation of nursing. By contrast, in the wake of NPM and consumer approaches, the British health system advances flexible regulation and provides new options for nursing (Burau, 1999; see also Allsop, 1999). A system like the National Health Service (NHS), widely seen as centralised, can therefore strengthen elements of decentralisation, whereas the German system fosters hierarchy. Similarly, in a regional British study Hughes and Griffiths (1999) were able to demonstrate that the decentralisation of health care and the centralised control of the NHS are parallel processes.

According to this research, decentralisation puts new demands on the state and may also enhance changes in the system of professions and further new professional projects, like community nursing. In addition, decentralisation is often linked to an improved user involvement in decision making. A decentralised health system therefore reinforces the need for negotiations on the balance of power and impacts in complex ways on the arrangement of stakeholders.

Regulatory power of culture and discourse in health care

Next to institutional regulation and macro–political change, informal modes of regulation play an important role in health care (Atkinson, 2002). According to Light, (1997, p 110), "health care systems are driven primarily by values, not by economic forces". A number of theoretical approaches are applied that move beyond institutional regulation, such as a Foucauldian concept of discourse, culture studies and concepts taken from new governance and the sociology of professions (see Chapter One, this volume). In particular, the concept of culture as outlined by Clarke (2004) and Newman (2005b) provides convincing examples that 'people, politics and public' are connected in more complex and dynamic ways.

This approach also directs attention towards the regulatory power of professionalism, in particular, the 'autonomy' of the medical profession and the shared public trust in the biomedical knowledge system. Although biomedical concepts grasp only specific aspects and caring needs, their explanatory power stretches over and shapes the entire health care system. However, the dominant values are currently undergoing significant change, which is most obvious in the area of public health. Saks describes the political development within the NHS as 'revolutionary':

> It continues to move away from an exclusive focus on the orthodox biomedical approach – centred on drugs and surgery – and gives greater recognition to socio-economic factors like unemployment and poor housing in relation to ill health, placing more stress on the consumer voice, public health, health promotion and health lifestyles. (1999, p 297)

With the growing significance of socioeconomic factors in health and health care systems, gender issues are also gaining ground. For the moment, this is most evident in the evaluation of managed care organisations (MCOs) in the US and the inclusion of women-centred approaches (Donaldson et al, 1996; Hoffman et al, 1997; McKinley et al, 2001). Nevertheless, as a result of political engagement of the WHO (WHO Euro, 2001) and the EU to introduce gender-mainstreaming policies, pressure is also increasing to include gender issues in European health systems too (Kuhlmann and Kolip, 2005). Subsequently, impulses for change not only stem from the health systems as such, but also, and to a great extent, from political pressure to promote gender equality.

As changes take place at different levels they do not necessarily unfold at the same time and can lead to tensions within a specific regulatory model, whether market, state or corporatist-oriented. This means that we cannot tell from an analysis of macro-political regulation of health systems precisely how impulses will be taken up at the level of organisations and the professions and what effects they will have on the quality of care.

Quality of care: from technological change to managerialism

Quality management is a cornerstone of the renewal of the public service sector and key to medical governance. The classic strategies of quality improvement via expansion of providers and services, new technologies and the specialisation of physicians no longer stand at unlimited disposal. The common answer to shortages of resources is managerialism. Two related but different strategies can be identified, namely rationalisation of the organisation and work (Donaldson et al, 1996; Campbell et al, 2000; Southern et al, 2002), and increased standardisation of care with performance indicators as measurements of quality (Exworthy et al, 2003). Increasingly, it is not simply a question of *what* is on offer, but *how* the services on offer are used in practice. These developments are summarised as a shift from structural to procedural change. The move from technological towards organisational and managerial change challenges the medical profession, but it also opens up new options to reassert power.

New demands on quality management and research

Quality of care is not defined in a uniform manner. In the biomedical quality debate, however, the definition of the US Institute of Medicine (IoM) is widely accepted. Quality, as defined here, is "the degree to which health services for individuals and populations increase the likelihood of successful health outcomes and are consistent with current professional knowledge" (Shine, 2000, p 2325). Research is dominated by the traditions of Donabedian (1988) and Cochrane (1972), which focus on clinical-epidemiological data. The Cochrane Reviews are highly influential in an international context, and RCTs count as a high level of proof in EBM (Sackett et al, 1997). Considerable extensions of quality indicators follow from a medical point of view, above all from the integration of user perspectives and EBM (Blumenthal, 1996).

However, to date it is hardly clear how, and using which indicators, the new goals of integration and coordination are to be examined (Southern et al, 2002). There is also a lack of indicators to measure public health and gender issues (Flood, 2004; Kuhlmann and Kolip, 2005), CAM therapies (Best and Glik, 2003), and quality at the level of individual providers (Gonen, 1999a). In addition, reliable quality indicators hardly exist for minor illness, which in primary care stands in the foreground (Campbell et al, 2000). Existing instruments do not, therefore, fit well with primary care, even though it is precisely this area that stands at the centre of the quality debate. The applied methods give priority to illness-related indicators and do not adequately grasp the increasing significance of prevention and health promotion.

What is taken into account is the new role of patients as consumers; their satisfaction is used to measure quality. Regarding the relevance and reliability of these measurements and the generally very positive results reported, a literature review on the subject concludes: "The measurement of patient satisfaction with traditional or new working models is generally unsophisticated" (Richards et al, 2000, p 192). This is confirmed by a Canadian study that does not find a significant correlation between patient satisfaction and the professional efficiency of nurses (Leiter et al, 1998). Thus, the relationship between quality and patient satisfaction is far too complex to be grasped with a linear model (see Chapter One, this volume). Similar problems can be seen in the indicator 'access to health care', which is increasingly used to evaluate quality of care (EUROPEP, 2002; HEDIS, 2002). Here, too, additional criteria are needed to assess *equity* of care and to make social inequalities – often related to gender – visible (Lindbladh et al, 1998).

Quality management primarily reacts to new demands in health care with the extension and standardisation of indicators (NHS CRD, 1999; EUROPEP 2002; HEDIS, 2002; Wensing et al, 2004), but does not overcome the blind spots of standardised measurements. The extended perspective of health reform models on social aspects of health and the organisation of care – such as coordination, teamwork and communication – are eventually reduced to biomedical-technological indicators, and lay perspectives consigned to the margins. This tendency is strengthened by the demand of proof of evidence of health care services. The increasing importance of economic criteria and the obligation to document and evaluate services lead to a prevalence of "quick fixes" (Grol et al, 2002, p 111). This means that only what is uncontested and easy to measure is taken into account. Subsequently, biomedical indicators may be reinforced as they enjoy the highest level of acceptance and have the most power to legitimate decisions (Harrison, 1998). Above all, quality of communication and the expert–lay relationship fall through this grid of standardisation (Campbell et al, 2000).

Given the increasing importance of EBM in health policy and practice, the revival of biomedical rather than social and system-based indicators may reinforce the power of the medical profession and a biomedical model of care. A further consequence is that no reliable research exists and there are no relevant indicators that prove, conclusively, that the assumed correlation between quality of care and managerial and organisational changes actually exists (Richards et al, 2000; Sicotte et al, 2002). The Cochrane Reviews are rather cautious in their assessment and have only been carried out so far for specific characteristics, namely coordination (Zwarenstein and Bryant, 2002), audits and reports (Currell et al, 2002; Thomson O'Brien et al, 2002a), guidelines (Thomas et al, 2002), interprofessional training (Zwarenstein et al, 2002), and continuous education and training (Thomson O'Brien et al, 2002b). There is an equal lack of knowledge on how to translate lay perspectives and subjective knowledge into quality indicators. We can conclude from existing research that seeing quality of care through the gaze of biomedicine and proceeding with new models of assessment along this avenue are not likely to enhance substantive changes in the epistemological fundament of health care or the power relations in this sector.

New models of quality assessment

Comparisons of health systems show that the effects of market-based steering tools and organisational changes do not necessarily impact negatively on the quality of care (Robinson and Steiner, 1998). The results do not, however, make it possible to draw any conclusions as to *which* characteristics of organisations lead to quality improvement or which have negative consequences. Here, approaches from the sociology of organisation and work provide more 'fine-tuned' indications and new data.

Comprehensive information comes from a Spanish study (Goni, 1999). This research asks how an instrument traditionally used in the private sector – with a teamwork-based organisation – impacts on effectiveness in health care. The author evaluates developments in Navarre, an autonomous region of Spain, where a teamwork philosophy was introduced into primary care in 1990. The study takes three different perspectives into account: the administration, the users and the workers. Results show that teams, where successful, can improve the quality of care. They "are a form of organizational design useful for improving performance in primary health care because insofar as they function properly, they achieve greater degrees of job satisfaction for the employees, greater perceived quality by the users and greater efficiency for the Administration" (Goni, 1999, p 107). Overall, this research somewhat modifies the vision that quality improvement and financial benefits can be achieved simultaneously, but it does support the thesis of quality improvement via integrative concepts and teamwork.

Findings from a Swedish study, which assessed the use of psychotropic drugs in 36 nursing homes, point in the same direction. The outcome measurements for drug use were set in relation to communication and cooperation between nurses and physicians. The relationship was assessed by two quality scores. Results show a positive correlation between quality of drug therapy and cooperation between physicians and nurses, including regular, multidisciplinary team discussions (Schmidt and Svarstadt, 2002).

These studies point to the significance of communication and flatter hierarchies in the workplace in order to improve quality of care. The results are confirmed in a Cochrane Review that demonstrates weak correlation between better coordination and cooperation of physicians and health professions, and a higher quality of care (Zwarenstein and Bryant, 2002). The authors call for systematic research, including qualitative studies, to more closely examine this correlation. Similarly, Canadian authors remind us, that "a first step is thus to better understand interdisciplinary collaboration before trying to link it to improved health" (Sicotte et al, 2002, p 994).

A number of studies in different countries – including Cochrane Reviews – have been carried out on changes arising from evaluation, auditing and clinical guidelines. Regarding guidelines, a Cochrane Review acknowledges only 'some evidence', to bring about effective changes in the process and outcome of care provided by professionals allied to medicine, but simultaneously warns against generalising the results (Thomas et al, 2002). For example, no effective correlation was found between the nursing report system and quality of care (Currell et al, 2002). The assessment of the audit system is also summarised with caution, as only "small to moderate but potentially worthwhile" effects were observed (Thomson O'Brien et al, 2002a). The influence of audits regarding the characteristics of teams working in the primary care of patients with diabetes was the subject of a qualitative British study (Stevenson et al, 2001). The authors identify four significantly correlated characteristics in the improvement of care for patients with diabetes:

> Success was more likely in teams in which: the GP or nurse felt personally involved in the audit; they perceived their teamwork as good; they had recognised the need for systematic plans to address obstacles to quality improvement;

and their teams had a positive attitude to continued monitoring of care. (2001, p 21)

Set against the backdrop of the Cochrane Reviews on auditing (Thomson O'Brien et al, 2002a) these results indicate that audits alone are not a strong indicator for quality of care, but that – under certain circumstances – they can have positive effects (see also Schepers and Casparie, 1999).

Taken together, the results indicate that new models of integrated care and organisational changes can improve quality of care to a certain extent, but such an outcome cannot be predicted owing to the complexity of influencing factors. Some positive effects can be expected from managerial tools – such as assessments, audits and guidelines – but even more from organisational change, in particular integrated models of care, teamwork and flatter hierarchies. Differentiated characteristics of improved quality are sustained quality management and cooperation and communication between occupational groups. Apart from structural change on the system level, organisational culture and changes on the micro-level of interaction contribute to the quality of care. These relationships lead to the notion of interprofessional collaboration and the role of organisations.

The organisation as the switchboard of change in health care

In the wake of managed care and marketisation, organisations become the switchboards of health care where macro-political regulatory incentives meet and are translated into practice. In particular, if primary care is to become the central pillar of health care systems, there is a need for fundamental change in the organisation (Shine, 2002) and composition of providers (Donaldson et al, 1996). Although governments respond to these demands in different ways, there is general consensus that provider networks should be given priority compared to the traditional solo-practices and the fragmentation of care (for instance, Batterham et al, 2002; Shine, 2002; Starfield and Shi, 2002; Dubois et al, 2006).

In the US we find a rapid increase in the number of MCOs, as well as growth in the areas of primary care, prevention and health promotion programmes (Donaldson et al, 1996). In Britain, new provider organisations, like the primary care groups (PCGs) and primary care trusts (PCTs), are emerging (Sheaff et al, 2004). These developments expand the circle of players way beyond the General Medical Council

(GMC), and give greater power to management, especially NHS managers (Allsop and Jones, 2006: forthcoming). New models of organisation can also be observed in continental Europe (Dent, 2003; Robelet, 2005) and in Canada (Coburn, 1999). In Germany, widespread debate on the monopoly of the medical profession in the delivery of ambulatory care and the demands of SHI funds for greater influence reflect similar tendencies, although no such fundamental structural changes have so far emerged (SVR, 2000/01, 2005); I will come back to this issue in the next chapter.

Key elements of organisational restructuring are teamwork and quality management. A statement by the IoM, for example, concludes, "teamwork is what counts [...] the current care systems cannot do the job. Changing systems of care is the only way to make the system better" (Shine, 2002, pp 10, 8). Donaldson and colleagues (1996) point out that, in primary care, it is not a question of *who* does something, but, above all, *how* this is being done. While the authors explicitly call for fundamental organisational changes, they conclude that a great variety of successful organisational models exist and that no recommendations can be given for any one model. In contrast to this, in Britain a specific organisational model is given preferred status in the form of PCGs – and more recently a merger of these groups to form PCTs – in order to establish an integrated system of care (Peckham and Exworthy, 2003).

Developments in the NHS bring about a "great organizational fluidity" (Light, 2001, pp 1178-9), which includes changes in the organisational structures in the direction of flatter hierarchies. Local professional networks increasingly monitor clinical practice. The innovative aspect is not simply the merger of providers but the tighter control and inclusion of physicians in a system of management. More recent studies from Britain highlight the problems and limitations of a network structure of governance. Fulop and colleagues studied PCGs in their second and third post-merger years and call for a more cautious approach on the likely gains: "Merger policy was based on simplistic assumptions about processes of organizational change that do not take into account the dynamic relationship between the organization and its context and between the organization and individuals within it" (2005, p 119; see Sheaff et al, 2004).

A closer look at teamwork provides further insights in these dynamics. Although there is very little empirical evidence on an overall innovation potential (Richards et al, 2000), the focus on teamwork offers possibilities for a more precise definition of terms like integration, cooperation and multidisciplinarity. For the main part, at the structural level this definition includes the occupational groups that comprise the team. On the process level it concerns the delegation of tasks within and between occupational groups, arrangements covering the organisation of work, cooperation and the competence and structure of decision making, as well as the cultural and micro-political organisational context. Apart from medical and epidemiological criteria, patient satisfaction is used as an indicator to measure outcome.

Multidisciplinary qualification and delegation of work

Multidisciplinary qualification is a vital characteristic of a PCT. In both the US and Britain the core of such teams appears to be developing in the direction of a combination of general care physicians and diverse health professions, which is expanded in nationally specific ways (Donaldson et al, 1996; Gonen, 1999b; Richards et al, 2000). With regard to the composition of professional qualifications in teams, we must take into account the very different qualification standards of health care workers that exist even within European countries (Dent, 2003; Theobald, 2004). Apart from national differences, multidisciplinary working groups offer a number of possibilities to delegate physicians' tasks to other professionals.

A review of Anglo-American studies shows that multidisciplinary teams carry out between 25% and 70% of all medical duties and that such groups can fulfil 20%-32% of outpatient care generally carried out by general practitioners (GPs) (Richardson et al, 1998). This means that the workload of physicians can be considerably reduced. Further British pilot studies point in the same direction (Gallagher et al, 1998; Jenkins-Clarke et al, 1998). Interestingly, physicians judge the possibilities of delegation to be lower than was shown in the pilot studies (Richardson et al, 1998). The delegation of tasks from physicians to other health professionals does, however, pose new problems concerning the re-negotiation of competencies and new workloads on health professions. In addition, delegation follows a gendered structure of work (Jenkins-Clarke et al, 1998) and this, in turn, could lead to new inequalities and new divisions of labour, especially in the highly unequal nursing sector (Dahle, 2003; Thornley, 2003).

Overall, investigations show that doctors' workloads can be reduced by around 50% by delegating certain primary care tasks to other health professionals. Moreover, these can then be further delegated to occupational groups, such as social workers, pharmacists, advisors or physicians' assistants. It is estimated that health assistants could carry out roughly 30% of the work of nurses (Richards et al, 2000). According to these findings, considerable potential for the rationalisation of health care lies in enabling health professionals and support workers to take over some work hitherto carried out by physicians or other higher status health professions. Accordingly, tensions between the economic logic of rationalisation and professional standards of care are embedded in the concept of delegation of work. This strategy is vulnerable to the ad hoc demands of the organisation and also to financial pressures from health policy. Delegation of work, therefore, may put new pressures on the health professions. It may reinforce hierarchies in some organisational contexts while improving career options and professionalisation in others.

Criteria of teamwork and barriers against integration and cooperation

Although multidisciplinary qualifications are an important prerequisite for a team, they are not strong indicators of effectiveness. Instead of delegation, which is based on an unequal distribution of power, effective teamwork calls for *integration* and a distribution of tasks appropriate to the qualifications and professional experience of the individuals involved (Richards et al, 2000; Elston and Holloway, 2001; Molyneux, 2001; Dubois et al, 2006). The conditions for successful integration are already set at the system level, as can be seen in health maintenance organisations (HMOs) in the US. This means that, in addition to the functions and the integration of team members, it is decisive whether the user has a choice between the physician and another health professional. Although most users still prefer the physician as primary care giver (Gonen, 1999c), the seemingly impermeable professional boundaries of medicine are becoming increasingly fluid, at formal levels, if users can choose between different professional groups.

With the softening of professional boundaries, the requirement arises for stricter regulation of work. Unclear roles, increasing workloads or lack of access to information lead to difficult conditions for teamwork (Richards et al, 2000). In contrast to this, improving communication is widely perceived as key to the effectiveness of teams. A survey based on interviews with British nursing teams explores further indicators of effectiveness, those of "understanding individual roles, appropriate use of skills, team involvement in decision-making, common objectives, developing shared protocols and innovation in practice" (Gerrish, 1999, p 373). Beyond that, interprofessional cooperation, consideration of patients' needs and the improvement of relations with GPs have a positive effect. Similar connectedness is manifest in multidisciplinary teams. The most important indicators of effective multidisciplinary teams are seen as clearly defined responsibilities, guidelines and assessments combined with programmes for improving quality (Richards et al, 2000; Sicotte et al, 2002). The formalisation of work can, therefore, nurture the cooperation and communication of diverse occupational groups (Sicotte et al, 2002).

However, an evaluation of a Spanish project highlights that change in the organisational culture does not automatically follow as a 'customary effect'; rather, satisfaction decreases significantly with the length of time an individual belongs to the organisation (Menarguez Puche and Saturno Hernandez, 1999). The assessment of a team concept in the Canadian health system – a system in which interdisciplinarity has been a guiding light over a period of many years – points in a similar direction: the introduction of interdisciplinarity and cooperation between occupational groups has delivered only moderate improvement in collaboration and reduction of conflict (Sicotte et al, 2002).

Barriers identified in the assessments of multiprofessional teams and the generally low levels of success achieved by new incentives for cooperation point to tensions and contradictions between the interests of different occupational groups. These contradictions are directly deposited in the new models of care; accordingly tensions may rise proportionate to the aggregate experience of the team. A major shortcoming of organisational restructuring and integrated caring concepts is a neglect of the tensions between the interests of the organisation and interest-based strategies of the various professions involved in the delivery of health care.

Professions in transition: old boundaries and new formations

New patterns of governance and new organisational models release considerable dynamics into professional areas. They bring about re-evaluations within medicine and new formations between the professions and occupations in the health sector. The hegemonic position of physicians is eroded and less assured in a formal manner when other professionals take on the same work but for less pay. With the expansion of health promotion and prevention, in addition to managerial tasks, qualifications and occupational groups that do not belong to the orthodox medical knowledge system are increasingly in demand. Not only is the circle of actors thereby expanded, but new criteria for decision making and new patterns of defining and legitimating quality of care are also introduced. Far-reaching changes in health policy and the organisation of work call for a 'future health workforce' (Davies, 2003) that better serves the demands on cooperation and integrated care.

Shifting relations within the system of professions

Although the dominance of the medical profession is coming under pressure to legitimise itself, especially in primary care, general medicine has achieved a rise in status within the profession. These developments are reported for the Anglo-Saxon systems (Fougere, 2001; Peckham and Exworthy, 2003), as well as for the US (Donaldson et al, 1996; Gonen, 1999c) and have recently become apparent in Germany as well (Kühn, 2001). One of the indicators used is to be found in employment statistics. The restructuring process increases the need for primary care doctors, whereas specialist treatment is steadily becoming more restricted, especially in the MCOs in the US. This restriction results in the return of specialists to general medicine where they meet with more favourable market conditions (Gonen, 1999b).

In different health systems we see that increase in status no longer necessarily follows the type of medical specialisation we know from classical pathways of professionalisation. This also leads to shifts, hardly analysed to date, in the gender arrangements of the medical profession. Indications can be drawn from a study that assessed the willingness of doctors in primary care in the US to innovate (Ubokudom, 1998). Viewed through a gender lens, the explored conditions that further positive attitudes on innovation – like working in group practices, lower level of specialisation and income, and younger age – more often apply to women than to men. Accordingly, the modernisation of health care and shifting gender relations need tackling as described elsewhere (Kuhlmann, 2001) with respect to the professionalisation of dentistry.

Shifting spheres of opportunity for female physicians may also be reinforced by consumerism. For example, a Dutch study highlights that the users of health care increasingly value the competence of female physicians, and this is also true for surgical and technological interventions, where confidence in women's abilities is generally expected to be lower (Kerssens et al, 1997). Consumerism may thus affect male and female professionals in different ways, and men and women may respond in different ways to the new demands on user involvement.

The enhanced shifts in the system of professions and the advance of new professional projects become even more evident when we look at the health professions. Primary care and the calls for teamwork and patient-centred care are the drivers for substantive change (Tovey and Adams, 2001). In Anglo-Saxon countries, nursing has long been more important in primary care. This has been accompanied by a huge increase in the number of nurses in Britain (Wilson, 2000; Dent, 2003). Gillam concludes that nurse practitioners are "paving the way for new forms of primary care management" (2003, p 196), and Saks (1999) highlights a new need for cooperation between GPs and community nurses. New opportunities for professionalisation are hereby open to nurses, especially in health promotion (Broadbent, 1998), but also regarding managerial work (Richards et al, 2000). In addition, a wide range of health care assistants, including the great majority of non-registered nurses, face new career opportunities (Thornley, 2003; similar developments are under way in Norway; see Dahle, 2003). Health reforms in the US have also raised the status of nurse practitioners (NPs), certified nurse midwives (CNMs) and physicians' assistants (PAs), all of whom work in most HMOs (Gonen, 1999b).

This entails a higher degree of diversity of health care providers and, subsequently, reinforces negotiations on competencies and the pay and grading systems (Thornley, 2003). Marketisation may accelerate the substitution of physicians and enhance significant shifts in the balance of power in health care, as the health professions are a cheaper workforce than doctors. Several studies confirm that this form of rationalisation does not necessarily reduce the quality of care. A follow-up study in the US, for instance, found after six and nine months no significant differences in the care delivered by physicians or nurses with respect to the medical outcome, the demand for services and patient satisfaction (Mundinger et al, 2000). Notably, already in the 1980s an investigation carried out by the US Office of Technology Assessment reached the same conclusion (Gonen, 1999b). These findings, however, take on new importance against the backdrop of increasingly tighter budgets. Similarly, in Britain it was shown that telephone advice by nurses was a safe and effective alternative to GP telephone advice and generally well accepted by patients (Dale et al, 1998).

A number of studies from different countries point out that a revaluation of primary care fosters the professionalisation of the health professions and favours new professional projects in areas with high proportions of women, in particular nursing. But it cannot be ignored that there may be an increase in occupational segments with low status that reinforces differences and inequalities within the nursing profession (Dahle, 2003; Theobald, 2003). A classic gendered pattern of professionalisation, therefore, needs reassessment and further differentiation.

Changing patterns of work

With high workloads, long working hours and on-call duties, occupational patterns in the medical profession generally correspond more closely to the work arrangements of men. This model, however, is undergoing significant change in all countries. As far as the medical profession in Britain is concerned, career paths are moving in the direction, formerly seen as typically female, of discontinuous career patterns, which are becoming the norm (Dowell and Neal, 2000). These 'portfolio careers' fit well with the changing conditions of health care systems that increasingly call for flexibility with regard to working hours, career patterns and work arrangements. Flexibility opens up chances for the organisation to use staff more effectively and cover the increased need for GPs (Young et al, 2001); this was also observed in nursing (Dahle, 2006: forthcoming).

Changing working patterns do not simply react to the demands of organisations; they are also an expression of more flexible gender arrangements and shifts in the work–life balance observed in different countries. Koninck and colleagues (1997) describe, for example, that women physicians in Canada plan their professional development and private lives in close proximity. In contrast to traditional developments, current tendencies show a slight rise in women's working hours, while men tend to work fewer hours. The working hours and career preferences of Dutch physicians in five specialist areas point in a similar direction. The authors report "that home domain characteristics, like children's age [...] did not predict a part-time preference for female, but for male [medical doctors]" (Heiligers and Hingstman, 2000, p 1235).

Therefore, the shifts in working and career patterns of health professionals arise, firstly, from the changed requirements and interests of the organisation, secondly, from an increase in the number of women in the workforce, and, thirdly, from the new working patterns of men. Results can probably not be generalised owing to differences in welfare states and incentive structures for employment market integration, especially of women with children (Lewis, 2002). Nevertheless, taken together, developments do point to a growing flexibility of gendered patterns of work that may be enhanced by organisational change.

Transforming professional identities

New demands on cooperation and teamwork act in opposition to the traditional medical culture of dominance and exclusion. Existing work arrangements reveal a persistent 'tribalism' of the medical profession, and at the same time new identities, which might promote a reduction of hierarchies (for instance, Löyttyniemi, 2001; Shine, 2002). While most research focuses on the medical profession, medical identities and the pride of autonomy are not the only barriers to modernisation. Historically, strong professional identities are to be found, above all, in nursing. A caring direction is often seen as the opposing pole to the biomedical–technological direction of the medical profession. Nursing identities, however, are currently undergoing considerable differentiation processes (Lucas and Bickler, 2000). They are more diverse and contradictory than medical identities, and resources for building occupational identity are more widely varied.

This also means that an assumed connection between the success of professional projects of nurses and changing priorities in health care – such as holistic, emotionally engaged concepts of care (Davies, 1996; Broadbent, 1998) – must be viewed more critically. Whether women will become change agents in the epistemological foundation of care cannot be concluded from their increasing physical presence in the field of health care (Riska, 2001b). At the same time new concepts of identity in nursing are described that may further collaboration. According to the results of a British survey of nurses, autonomy and teamwork stand in positive correlation. Contrary to classic expectations, autonomy and teamwork do not necessarily conflict (Rafferty et al, 2001).

In addition to the medical and nursing professions, with the increasing significance of managerialism another group of professionals enters into the system of professions. Most importantly, this group, of health managers, follows another normative orientation than that of the traditional health professions (McConnell, 2002). The advance of managerialism in health care releases tensions that are not studied with respect to their dynamics in the system. Economic concepts of 'rational choice' and a utilitarian logic are commonly set in contrast to the altruistic norms of medicine and the caring values of nursing. Management is a far less homogeneous group than medicine, and professional boundaries are less important for the creation of hierarchies here. This group is more strongly characterised by organisational than professional culture.

Results show that diverse and sometimes conflicting identities do not only exist between the medical and the health professions, and tensions do not follow one single line of division. Different normative orientations are coming together within the new organisational models of teamwork that do not easily merge to a new identity of primary care workers. Existing results do *not* point to a loss of the identity building importance of the professions but to an increasing diversity of resources with which identities – more hybrid ones – can be constructed. A Canadian study highlights that the jurisdiction of professional boundaries and 'professional wars', as described by Abbott (1988), are still highly relevant today. What is new, however, is that *in addition* to this culture of conflict and exclusion, new logic and new values of interprofessional cooperation are in the process of emerging. The authors conclude that "both logics, competitive and collaborative, are thus present at the same time and influence collaborative service delivery" (Sicotte et al, 2002, p 999).

Professional identities are not necessarily an obstacle to cooperation, but they can be activated and employed as lines of demarcation when it comes to the jurisdiction of interests. Similarly, gender provides a resource for the jurisdiction of professional status. However, so-called female professions can adopt male-connoted identities, such as hardiness (Riska and Wrede, 2003). Men in the professions can take up – and are increasingly forced to do so by market conditions – working patterns hitherto reserved for women, especially women with caring responsibilities. Gender thus remains a powerful order of professions but it is no longer congruent with women's quotas and sex category.

Dynamics of organisational change and flexible professional boundaries

This exploration of key concepts of restructuring and areas of change in different health systems shows that modernisation processes bring about a new need for regulation and more complex models of governance (Allsop, 1999; Allsop and Jones, 2006: forthcoming). Governing health care occurs more as a network structure into which a multitude of regulatory impulses flow, thus releasing new dynamics in health care. Put in terms of new institutionalism, regulation follows a 'loose coupling' of formal rules and professional practice (Dent, 2003). Organisations and professions are key dimensions to exploring the ties and tensions, and the power relations of this network structure of governance and its contribution to quality management.

Organisational restructuring and professional interests are interconnected in a way that enhances ongoing dynamics (Davies, 2003; Nancarrow and Borthwick, 2005; McKee et al, 2006). This is clearly illustrated in teamwork, which leads to a differentiation rather than a collaborative health workforce – as would be functional for teamwork. It has rather a strengthening than a levelling effect on professional identities. However, new professional projects manifest new strategies, which cannot be grasped in the categories of classical professionalisation. We find both more flexible professional boundaries as well as the emergence of new ones – for example, in nursing (Dahle, 2006: forthcoming) – and a revaluation of professional segments as seen in medicine. More importantly, organisational change and the upgrading of primary care foster professionalisation of the wide range of health occupations and professions and the integration in the system of care. These processes, in turn, enhance changes in the gendered division of labour and working arrangements.

The aim of this chapter has been to explore global trends and key dimensions of change. The strongest predictor for change seems to be the introduction of primary care and the strengthening of integrated caring models based on teamwork and cooperation between and within professions. Restructuring the system of care and the provider organisations enhances various dynamics in the division of labour and quality of care, and poses the highest level of challenge to the professions, especially physicians. Compared to this, the dynamics of managerialism and scientific-bureaucratic measurements, as well as improved user participation, are weaker and more related to changes within the medical profession. The potential for sustainable change, however, may increase when these strategies are expanded to the entire health workforce, and the demands of consumers gain ground at all levels of regulation.

THREE

Remodelling a corporatist health system: change and conservative forces

International calls for the coordination and integration of provider services, and participation of consumers, are echoed in Germany. In particular, the 2004 Health Modernisation Act paved the way for organisational change and new forms of managerialism and provider control. This chapter outlines the conditions and dynamics of modernising health care in a conservative corporatist welfare system, with particular emphasis on interoccupational change. By combining structure and policy, and static and dynamic analysis, it brings the reflexive nature of change in health into focus. Starting with an overview of the characteristics of the German health system, the major regulatory incentives of health reform Acts from the 1990s onwards are discussed; strategies are specified for quality management and new organisational models. This is followed by information on changes in the occupational structure. Putting the focus on the medical profession as a key player, physiotherapists and surgery receptionists are studied in order to grasp interoccupational dynamics. The findings highlight the coexistence of innovation and conservatism. Corporatism has not been replaced but is transformed and supplemented with elements from new governance. These developments put new challenges on the professions, and also new demands on the state to govern what has become a more hybrid network of public law institutions.

Regulatory framework: change and corporatist conservatism

Corporatism and federalism are key elements of health politics and a particular approach to policy making in Germany (Schwartz and Busse, 1997). Within the corporatist system of governance the state provides the framework for a network of public law institutions (Moran, 1999) and integrates federal interests by drawing on an extensive legal framework (Social Code Book V). The state hands over rights and responsibilities for service delivery to the corporatist self-governing institutions, which have mandatory membership and the right to negotiate contracts and raise their own financial resources. SHI funds and physicians' associations are the 'core' of corporatist regulation. This structure is especially strong in ambulatory care, although this model is increasingly expanding to the hospital sector.

The Federal Association of SHI Physicians represents the interests of doctors on the provider side and is simultaneously a public law institution. This double function is the Achilles heel of Germany's health system and key to understanding corporatist regulation and the power of the medical profession. The medical profession is strongly self-regulated by statutory chambers established at federal, regional and local levels, and this also applies to dentists and pharmacists. Other health occupations and CAM therapists are not included in this system of professional chambers. Nor are these groups represented in the regulatory bodies, although they have been undergoing change since the 1990s and markedly extended with the 2004 Health Modernisation Act. "Nurses, midwives, physiotherapists and other groups are not considered to be professionals in the legal sense" (European Observatory on Health Care Systems, 2000, p 27). The system is highly physician-centred and biased towards curative and acute care: it is characterised by a high density of physicians, nurses, and hospital beds, short, if any, waiting lists and a community-centred provision of care.

Physicians are the market-shaping service provider and simultaneously wield considerable influence in all regulatory bodies. Most importantly, the physicians' and dentists' associations have the corporatist monopoly and the legal obligation to deliver and secure ambulatory care. They are legally bound to guarantee service (*Sicherstellungsauftrag*). This means that sickness funds and others are not allowed to provide ambulatory care. The SHI physicians' association prospectively negotiates the health care budget and then distributes the global budget among its members according to a defined fee system (European Observatory on Health Care Systems, 2000). This powerful position of physicians is, however, coming under increasing critique. A number of policy initiatives aim to weaken this monopoly by allowing for more flexible contracting and the provision of ambulatory surgery by hospitals.

The individual practice and the independent professional – specialist and generalist – are the dominant organisational forms in ambulatory care, upheld by a fragmentation of hospital and ambulatory care. The ambulatory sector is clearly dominated by solo practices (73%). The proportion of group surgeries is growing only slowly – between 1993 and 2000 by around 3% – and in absolute numbers, generalists (including the former category *Praktische Ärzte*) are even less likely than specialists to work in a group practice (author's own calculations, source KBV, 2000, p A33). Furthermore, we find deficiencies – or a sheer absence – of transparency, evaluation of services, comprehensive data, standards of care and clinical guidelines, as well as inefficient quality management and weak user participation (Moran, 1999; SVR, 2000/01, 2003). However, improving quality of care and transparency of services is at the top of the political agenda, and more active user participation also makes progress.

The SHI funds are the second key player in the corporatist system. They traditionally act as the representatives of the user interests, and this role is democratically legitimised via elections of the regulatory bodies of the funds. They are self-administered, non-profit organisations and represent 90% of the population. The remaining 10% is privately insured and represented by the organisation of private insurers (KBV, 2000, p G1). While there have been numerous SHI funds, since the 1990s health policy has attempted to merge different funds (European Observatory on Health Care Systems, 2000); numbers have been slimmed down from about 400 SHI funds in 2000 to about 290 in 2005. SHI care accounts for the lion's share of health care expenditure (57%; StatBA, 2003a). Most CAM therapies are excluded from the SHI system, although there are some overlaps, for instance, in physiotherapeutic care. State interest in the control of providers and standardisation of these services is consequently low.

In keeping with the Bismarckian or social insurance-based model, Germany's health care system is based on a concept of social solidarity. Equity, access to health care and the freedom to choose a provider are highly prized cultural values embedded in the system of Statutory Health. The SHI system is funded by equal contributions from employers and individuals. The coupling of social insurance contributions and salary makes health care expenditure highly visible (Moran, 1999) but, at the same time, public control is limited with regard to funding and provision of service. A falling income rate and high levels of unemployment in Germany directly impact on funding, thereby exerting constant pressure on the government to reduce expenditure (Blank and Burau, 2004).

The Federal Committee of Physicians and Health Insurance Funds is the most important public law institution that negotiates issues of SHI care. With the 2004 Health Modernisation Act stakeholder regulation is expanded and consumer representatives are included for the first time in the most important regulatory body, which is now called the Federal Committee. In addition, the Advisory Council for the Evaluation of the Department of Health Care System (SVR) can be viewed as a hybrid structure between institutional regulation and political discourse. Recent reviews make strong demands for quality improvement, consumer participation and cooperation of providers (SVR, 2003, 2005), thereby furthering a 'global' policy discourse of restructuring.

Besides institutional regulation and policy discourse, cultural values impact on the health policy process. The health political culture is shaped by a "strong tradition of voluntarism, self-help and family support, embedded in Roman Catholic teaching and the idea of subsidiarity" (Blank and Burau, 2004, p 42). At the same time, 'familialism' (Dent, 2003) is described as an important barrier to the professionalisation of nursing and women's career chances, and therefore relevant for all health occupations with an overall high proportion of women. Gender asymmetry is embedded in all health care systems but impacts in various ways according to national differences in the 'gender contract' (Siim, 2000). In the German welfare system conservative elements of both a gender contract and health political culture intersect, and provide another source of conservatism and stability in addition to institutional regulation. However, stability is on the wane and increasingly challenged by changes in the family structure and women's labour market participation.

Conservative forces also derive from the historically developed principles of citizen *rights* on comprehensive health care and the freedom to choose a provider, as well as the medical profession's normative claims for autonomy. Accordingly, both users and dominant providers of health care accentuate cultural values, which limits the scope of health policy to advance managerial strength and organisational coherence in health care. Attempts by the government to enhance organisational change and improve provider control may thus face multiple barriers and hardly predictable transformations on their way into practice. The following sections outline how health policy responds to new demands and how new policies translate into changes in health care and the professions.

Transforming a network of public law institutions

A series of reform Acts from the 1990s onwards bear witness to strong pressure to innovate the health system. Striking advantages of compulsory health insurance for all citizens, easily accessible health services, and solidarity and responsiveness of the Bismarckian system go hand in hand with fundamental weaknesses of the system (SVR,

2000/01, 2003). According to criteria used in a WHO comparison of about 190 health systems, Germany is in 25th place. The outcome and performance indicators are weak (Busse and Schlette, 2004) despite Germany's high placing regarding health care expenditure (European Observatory on Health Care Systems, 2000; StatBA, 2003b, p 15). Major critique focuses on a high fragmentation of providers and services combined with an orthodox curative orientation and a physician-centred system. The recent reviews of the Advisory Council (SVR, 2003, 2005) highlight the need for improved coordination of provider services, quality management and consumer participation.

Despite a wide range of system weaknesses, cost containment is the most powerful policy driver for change. The US strategy of cost control – managed competition – was used to point the way to restructuring (Kühn, 1997). The introduction of free choice of sickness funds for all citizens and market competition within the SHI system, legally fixed budgets on the provider side, exclusion of several health services from SHI care and increasing co-payment of patients bear witness to these steering impulses, which were strengthened as the 1990s progressed (for an overview see Deppe, 2000; European Observatory on Health Care Systems, 2000). Marketisation and the dominance of cost containment reflects a 'global' turn towards neoliberalism in health care systems (Coburn, 1999). However, since the beginning of the 21st century, patterns from NPM and state regulation have been gaining ground and policy goals extended. The main stages of the modernisation of ambulatory care are given in Table 3.1.

Characteristic of new policies is that they are directed primarily at a short-term reduction of costs and addressed almost exclusively to the medical profession and the SHI funds. The politics of cost containment do not grasp the key problem of health economy, namely the falling income rate and demographic change (Blank and Burau, 2004). They also fail to respond to the wide range of new demands, and do not systematically touch on the system deficits of health care. The health reform Acts of the 1990s have fallen short of the targets with regard to both cost-containment and quality of care (Schöffski and Schulenburg, 1997; SVR, 2000/01, 2003). The financial efficiency of new models of care, such as disease management programmes (DMPs), is also viewed with scepticism (Gerst et al, 2005), and various attempts to further organisational change have largely failed (Häussler et al, 2001). At the same time, the politics of marketisation enhanced change in the system of SHI funds, in particular a growing merger of funds and a move away from bureaucratic towards more flexible and service-oriented organisations (Bode, 2003). However, these

Table 3.1: Health reform Acts from the 1990s onwards: major changes and policy goals

Health reform Acts	Changes ↔ policy goals
Health Structure Acts 1992-95 *Seehofer Reform*	Free choice of sickness funds; limitation of the number of SHI physicians and dentists and economic feasibility assessment; pilot projects to introduce a gatekeeper system; a more flexible system of tariffs or case fees replaces fixed budgets for SHI physicians ↔ to shift the balance of power towards the SHI funds; to upgrade general care; to strengthen competitive elements in the SHI system
Health Insurance Contribution Rate Exoneration Act 1996 Statutory Health Insurance Restructuring Act 1997	Fees fixed for each group of physicians; softening of the principle of collective contracting; introduction of 'tailored services' (*IgeL Leistungen*; Krimmel, 2000) that are excluded from SHI care; limitation of SHI care, particularly in dental care and rehabilitation ↔ to strengthen competitive elements within the medical profession and between physicians and SHI funds; to increase the co-payment of users
Health Reform Act 2000	Competitive structure extended; framework agreements on integrated care (Social Code Book V § 140d); pilot projects and contracts on structural change (Social Code Book V §§ 63ff, § 73a. § 140b) ↔ to facilitate organisational change; to merge physicians into networks; to upgrade general medical care; to further increase co-payment of users
DMPs 2002	Introduction of standardised programmes for some chronic illnesses, namely CHD, diabetes mellitus type II and breast cancer; advancement of clinical guidelines, EBM, quality assurance; inclusion of user representatives in the regulatory boards; mandatory evaluation; limitation of free choice of providers, but voluntary participation of both providers and users ↔ to change the organisation of care and to move towards a gatekeeper system; to strengthen general medical care; to set up targets and standards; to improve transparency of services and the control of providers; to improve patient information; to expand regulatory bodies; to improve cooperation between physicians; to strengthen the position of SHI funds
Health Modernisation Act 2004	Expansion of stakeholder regulation and transformation of the key regulatory body of SHI funds and physicians' associations into the Federal Committee; inclusion of user representatives in the policy process; quality management; legal rules on continuous education of physicians; increased co-payment of the users; strengthening of general medical care and preventive care; financial incentives for providers and users towards a gatekeeper system ↔ to facilitate organisational change; to improve user participation, control of providers and quality management; to increase competition within the medical profession; to strengthen the position of SHI funds; to limit free choice of providers and specialist care

developments also provoked unintended dynamics in the SHI system, for instance growing social inequality through increased co-payment of the users and exclusion of services from SHI care (StatBA, 2003b; Streich, 2003), and an increasing pressure on physicians to act according to financial interests (Kuhlmann, 1998, 1999).

While it is true that the reform Acts were less successful than some had hoped, they nevertheless opened the way for other important changes and future prospects (Glaeske et al, 2001). Health policy is increasingly turning to individual providers, instead of collective contracting of the SHI physicians' associations, and expanding their options of choice with regard to reimbursement. This strategy provides new resources to shift the balance of power away from the physicians' associations and to engage SHI funds in the steering goals of the state. This attempt reflects a salient interest of the state that is as old as Statutory Health itself. The strengthening of SHI funds was especially pronounced in times of economic crisis, like the Weimar Republic, and lost ground in the 'golden age' of medicine in the postwar period. Given the 21st century's problems of cost containment in the health care system, the strategy is facing revival once again.

The reform Acts confirm that a classic pattern of solving financial problems through simply shifting the balance of power *within* the stakeholder arrangement continues to dominate health policy. At the same time, policy goals are becoming more diverse, particularly reflecting a need for quality management, new models of care and user participation. The following sections review a dominant thesis of 'decorporisation' (Stillfried, 2000) and turn attention towards the *transformations* of corporatism enhanced through patterns from new governance.

Improving quality management and public control

The politics of cost containment and marketisation shape the debate on quality of care and public control of providers. Target setting, documentation and evaluation of health care are underdeveloped areas in the German system. In 2001 the Advisory Council stated: "the lack of positive incentives for the establishment and implementation of quality measures. [...] there are no incentives in the health care system to stimulate competition among health care providers that is based on the factor of quality" (SVR, 2000/01, p 71). Moreover, the other side of the coin has also been neglected, namely, the provision of a system of sanctions against those who provide poor quality of care (Sauerland, 2001). According to the Advisory Council no effective and dependable public system of quality control existed for services in the health care sector (SVR, 2000/01, pp 74-5).

Given the situation, the medical profession has developed its own strategies. Community-based, loosely linked working groups and the quality circles of physicians rapidly sprung up. Quality circles are based on voluntary membership, self-regulation and the shared interests of members. In general, they are registered with the physicians' chambers and typically comprise working groups of eight to 15 physicians. Consequently, there is wide variation in the structure and efficiency of such quality circles, and their contribution to quality improvement is not evaluated. Characteristically, while quality circles individually lead to the improved qualification of some physicians, they have no public control function. Where regulation does exist, it embodies the right of self-regulation of physicians. It is interesting to note, however, that the Advisory Council sees the tasks of quality circles also in "medical controlling based on quality indicators" (SVR, 2000/01, p 74). This statement brings into view that a classic strategy of assuring quality through highly qualified physicians is supplemented by new forms but not transferred to public control via independent actors and institutions.

Although quality circles do not indicate a change towards tighter public control, they are proof of a cultural change in the medical profession and a new willingness to review individual practice. After an initial phase of scepticism and rejection, the medical profession embraced the language of EBM and quality management. Numerous training courses and certificates offered by the physicians' academies – the professions' own body of qualification – bottom-up initiatives and a rapidly expanding academic debate indicate that the medical profession has incorporated new forms of managerial regulation (Robra, 2005). With regard to other health occupations the impact of new patterns of quality management has been much weaker, and effects on professionalisation less clear.

Signs have recently begun to emerge that the state is now more willing to exercise its power in order to improve the control of physicians (Di Luzio, 2004). For example, since 2004 continuing education of physicians is defined by law, and a national Institute of Quality and Efficiency in Health Care has been established. This institute is becoming a signifier of a new pattern of institutional control beyond the classical corporatist arrangement. In the same vein, in 2004 the Federal Ministry of Health introduced the office of a patient representative in the federal government. In addition, almost all sickness funds improved patient information and introduced new forms of user involvement, such as call centres (Wöllenstein, 2004). At present, the quality of these services is not monitored and competencies and qualification of staff not defined.

These developments are evidence of the advancement of state-centred elements of governance and public control. At the same time, they reproduce classical elements of corporatist regulation in Germany, namely the strong position of the medical profession. For example, the Institute of Quality and Efficiency in Health Care is headed by a physician and focuses on biomedical issues of health care. The intention, once again, is not to include the whole range of providers of health care services – or service users – in the system of quality management and control.

A physician-centred and biomedically biased system of control impacts in different ways on the various occupational groups and areas of health care, but provides most opportunity for the medical profession to resist tighter regulation in order to protect market interests and exclude other providers from the SHI system. For example, the integration of acupuncture into Statutory Health was the subject of negotiations within the Federal Committee in 2004 but reimbursement was rejected. Notably, physicians increasingly offer acupuncture as a service that patients have to pay for themselves. Subsequently, SHI regulation of this service runs contrary to the interests of the medical profession as fees would be fixed and markets more regulated. This example highlights that the German model of quality management in general runs contrary to public control and stronger regulation of the entire spectrum of health care services. A policy discourse on tighter provider control and the introduction of elements from 'medical governance' (Gray and Harrison, 2004) does not tell, therefore, whether and how medical power actually is reduced.

Changing the organisation of providers

A number of pilot projects, initiated at the end of 1990s, are based on concepts from managed care (Table 3.1). The German version of managed care fits the description of a 'loosely coupled system' (Weick, 1976) aimed at organisational change. Managed care is embraced by sickness funds above all as an alternative provider model. Office-based generalists are to act as gatekeepers regarding appointments with specialists and clinical treatment, thereby reducing SHI expenditure. Characteristic is a wide diversity of forms of organisation and wide room for manoeuvre for corporatist actors in shaping the pilot projects.

This is especially visible when we look at the new forms of contracting introduced with the 2000 reform Act (Table 3.1).

If we count every single agreement that deals with better coordination and cooperation of providers or with quality management in any way, for 2002 we find a total of 21 contracts on pilot projects and 16 on structural change (author's own calculations, source: KBV, 2002a). Notably, some contracts relate to only one sickness fund – among about 400 in Germany (European Observatory on Health Care Systems, 2000) – or one single illness, in particular, diabetes. Furthermore, contracts are in place in only 14 of the 23 regions of SHI physicians' associations (author's own calculations, source: KBV, 2002a). If we take into account only those contracts that deal, strictly speaking, with the networks of physicians and integrated care, the number falls significantly. According to a publication from the Federal Association of SHI Physicians for 2002 we find 25 contracts (Tophoven, 2003, p 87).

We see that the subject of integrated care approaches has only been raised by some SHI funds in a few regions of Germany, and only for certain illnesses. In addition, considerable problems emerge in the management of new networks (Lingenfelder and Kronhardt, 2003), which sometimes disintegrate after a short time. Overall, existing investigations show that the financial success of networks is, at best, slight. An important piece of mosaic in the German managed care scenario – the pilot projects and contracts on structural change – has thus failed to materialise (Häussler et al, 2001). The state provides the legal framework and financial incentives for integrated caring models, but it does not directly intervene in the organisation of providers. Overall, the various initiatives lack managerial strength, and the process of change is not adequately monitored.

Both weaknesses are addressed with the introduction of DMPs, the most concrete step taken to date to adjust integrated models of care to German conditions (SVR, 2003; Table 3.1, this volume). The association with a risk compensation scheme aligns the DMPs to a pattern of health policy governed by economic goals (BMG, 2002, p 1). However, the new programmes move beyond cost containment and raise the need for new patterns of procedural regulation, performance indicators and new regulatory boards (Schmacke, 2002; Pfaff et al, 2003).

They have given rise, first and foremost, to the clearest shift to date in the arrangement of public law institutions. Second, the network structure of corporatist actors is becoming more flexible and interests more diverse. And third, it promotes cooperation within the medical profession, which, in turn, reinforces the need to negotiate professional boundaries and responsibilities. Furthermore, and equally important, the new programmes extend the range of orthodox medicine, and attempt to improve patient information and participation. This raises the requirement for new demands and competencies that go beyond biomedical care, for instance nutritional advice, psychological counselling and physical exercise. The enhanced flexibility of regulation opens windows of opportunity to include new actors and new performance indicators of quality, for example gender-sensitive measurements (Kuhlmann and Kolip, 2005).

In conclusion, health policy provides a number of new options for organisational change and more flexible patterns of network governance; the state increasingly demonstrates a new willingness to exercise power. However, these demonstrations do not necessarily incite substantial changes in the power relations of the corporatist arrangement. Although the DMPs turn the tide towards tighter regulation, a characteristic lack of managerial strength of restructuring in Germany is reproduced: the state does not take over the task of coordination and fails to integrate new occupational fields and professional groups. This, in turn, creates a vacuum, which is filled almost exclusively by the most powerful actor: the medical profession and its network initiatives of bottom–up governance.

Most of these networks are established at community level and operate outside the legally defined framework of pilot projects and contracts, often opting to operate under the status of a registered charity (Nagel, 2002). Accordingly, they are not interested in contracts with sickness funds (Tophoven, 2003). Interestingly, the networks of physicians sprang up and spread very rapidly after the state-driven initiatives based on financial rewards were seen to have failed. No reliable data are available on the organisational structure and working patterns of physicians' networks; it is not even known how many networks there are. This is a further sign of weakness in the system of corporatist governance. The state does not take over the task of monitoring new organisational models but leaves this in the hands of SHI funds and the medical profession.

A questionnaire study recently carried out by a regional SHI physicians' association provides some data on doctors' pros and cons for networks (Nagel, 2004). Political motives, especially to strengthen professional interest vis-à-vis SHI funds, were by far the most common reason given in this survey. Personal and professional contacts with colleagues and improving the quality of care featured in middle field, and economic interests at the bottom of this ranking. A previous evaluation of one network in a northern region of Germany showed similar results (Nagel, 2002). The author emphasises that the strengthening of professional interests related to networks does not necessarily go against the interests of physicians' associations. Results of this study indicate significant shifts in the medical culture of 'autonomy'. At the same time, 'independence from management' and 'self-determination' remain strong values – more emphasised by specialists than generalists (Nagel, 2004) – that may lead to negative attitudes to networks. Furthermore, professional interests are a weaker motive for network membership for the youngest generation of practitioners (Nagel, 2004).

The power of networks to enhance sustainable change in the organisation of care may be limited owing to decentralisation and a lack of formalisation and stability; the contribution to quality improvement also remains weak (SVR, 2003). However, the impact of networks goes far beyond organisational change. Networking unites very different – and even contradictory – motives. This makes the networks an unknown quantity in the area of governance, especially against the backdrop of a growing dissatisfaction with the politics of professional associations (Brechtel, 2001). Results also point to more hybrid pattern of governance and the key role of the professions in shaping and transforming policy goals.

Changes in the professions: uneven developments towards modernisation

The previous sections have shown that the professions may accelerate dynamics that are not fully predictable from policies and institutional regulation. In accordance with the physician–centred nature of health policy, the focus has been on the medical profession. This section takes a closer look at occupational conditions and change in other sections of the health workforce, which is particularly linked to changes in gender relations and the working patterns of women. I would like to call in mind the importance of the health sector in the labour market, especially for women. While women represent 44% of the total workforce, their proportion in the health sector in 2002 was 72%; in contrast to men, participation of women in the health labour market in general is on the increase (StatBA, 2004), and this also applies to the medical profession (BLK, 2004).

The three selected groups represent different positions and power resources in the health sector (see Introduction, this volume). Physicians, as the dominant group, represent an archetype of a profession with high status and power over other occupational groups. This profession is characterised by a gendered occupational structure and employment patterns that are based on a 'male' work pattern. Physiotherapy represents a middle-of-the-field health occupation, and a professional project of a formerly female occupation between health care services subordinated to physicians and CAM practitioners. Physiotherapists exemplify the growing importance of CAM therapies between SHI funding and privately paid care (Dixon et al, 2003). Physiotherapy is also an example of a group of independent therapists, not integrated into a surgery setting, but who generally take instructions from a physician. Surgery receptionists rank lowest among the health occupations with low income and status, and clear subordination to physicians. This is a classical female occupation where we find the persistence of sex segregation, and one which does not provide any career tracks. With respect to numbers, surgery receptionists are the largest single group in ambulatory care (GBE, 1998a, 2005). They fit the category of health support workers; they are responsible for tasks that are usually carried out by low-status nurses, nursing assistants or PAs in other health systems.

The impact of policy changes is not adequately monitored, and consequently no reliable data exist on the occupational structure; for instance, the Health Reports for Germany (GBE, 1998a, 1998b, 2005) provide only very rough data. Data are worst when it comes to the health occupations and their services (European Observatory on Health Care Systems, 2000; Scharnetzky et al, 2004). The results presented in the following sections are based mainly on my own calculations of statistics from the Federal Association of SHI Physicians, and additional information from various sources, including expert estimations. The analysis highlights the impact of the 1990s reforms driven by economic logic, and in some cases tendencies of the reform Act in 2000; more recent changes are studied empirically and presented in Part II of this volume. Starting with an overview of the occupational situation, changing market conditions and interprofessional developments provide the connecting link between the three groups.

Medical profession: defence of status and increasing differentiation

Physicians have an overwhelmingly high social status and belong to the "peak earners among academics" (GBE, 2002, p 8.7). They face the advantages of state-regulated and limited access to medical schools and markets, in particular SHI care. Of the total of 291,000 physicians, 43% work in ambulatory care; 90% of these are office-based SHI physicians, 6% are employees in surgeries, and 4% treat privately insured patients and are not part of the SHI system (source: KBV, 2000, p A1). SHI physicians thus represent 96% of all physicians working in ambulatory care and serve as a basis in the following analysis.

While at the beginning of the 1990s falling market power of the medical professions is described as a result of increasing numbers of physicians and growing competition (Alber, 1992), a turning point was reached in the mid-1990s. The number of physicians entering the register started to fall for the first time (source: KBV, 2000, p J3); the number of SHI physicians increased very slightly (source: KBV, 2000, p A8); and the unemployment rate was markedly low (4%; source: KBV, 2000, p H3). Added to this, the demographic structure of the medical profession indicates improved employment options for the younger physicians (BÄK, 1997). It is interesting to note that the loss of attractiveness of a medical career applies only to male physicians, while the number of women steadily increases (BLK, 2004, p 11). These trends are reinforced as the 21st century proceeds. Meanwhile, a shortage of doctors, in particular in the eastern *Länder* of Germany, and worries about 'feminisation' of medicine are a concern of the profession.

The favourable situation in the employment market comes up against the state's regulatory attempts to contain cost, which results in falling incomes for physicians. At the same time, new services, not reimbursed via the SHI system, such as preventive programmes and CAM, open up new market segments, and overall health care expenditure continues to rise (source: KBV, 2000, p K5). Patient co-payment is also increasing, and the 'tailored services' (Table 3.1) generate extra income for physicians, which lies outside public control. We can therefore assume growing differentiation within the medical profession. Statistics indicate a wide and increasing variation of income (source: KBV, 2000, p D11), and in this respect, the politics of competition actually provoke change in the profession.

The effects of health policies are less striking when it comes to restructuring. Given that market conditions have a considerable influence on whether and how the medical profession accepts restructuring, pressure for change seems to be moderate at this level, and does not affect all groups in the same way. Data indicate that the new regulatory models aimed at the upgrading of general care and limitation of specialists have not, so far, led to any noteworthy shift within the profession. Between 1996 and 2000 – when new policies CAMe into force (Table 3.1) – the proportion of generalists (including *Praktische Ärzte*) decreased by 2.5% but the number of specialists rose (source: BÄK, 1997, p 12; KBV, 2000, p A8). Furthermore, generalists make up 39% of SHI physicians but receive only 32% of the total budget (source: KBV, 2000, p D8). Generalists in the western part of Germany have had a slightly lower loss of revenue, but in the new *Länder* they have clearly higher losses than the specialists (source: KBV, 2000, pp D9-10). On average, specialists come off better than generalists with respect to numbers and income, but tendencies are not uniform.

Set against the backdrop of the lower prestige associated with general medicine we can observe a very slow approximation of the two professional groups, although not a fundamental re-evaluation. Nonetheless, specialists and generalists act within two very different paradigms. While specialists are fighting to retain their status and some segments are having to accept regional losses, the aims of health policy to upgrade general care can be used to improve the status of this group.

Data indicate that a 'core' of medical professionalisation – the division and hierarchy between generalists and specialists – is resistant to change, while gender relations – a further characteristic of medical professionalisation – show the clearest shifts today. Among first-term medical students, women are now in the majority, with 64% (BLK, 2004, p 11). An increase of women in the profession is consistent overall with regard to both qualifications and in the occupational field (KBV, 2000, p J7; BLK, 2004). What is remarkable here is that the number of male doctors declined for the first time in 2001 while the number of women doctors continued to increase (Marburger Bund, 2002). With a proportion of 36%, women are more highly represented under generalists than under specialists (31%) (source: KBV, 2000, p A14). Developments indicate a clear shift towards more equal ratios of men and women, but at the same time, gender inequality persists – borne out, for instance, by a lower ratio of self-employment (Blättel-Mink and Kramer, 2006: forthcoming), the lower income of female practice owners (ZM, 2004a) and the lower participation and status of women in the associations (KBV, 2002b; Marburger Bund, 2002).

The innovative aspect is that health policies favour an occupational field with higher proportions of women compared to the profession as a whole. The classic relationship between low prestige of a professional segment and high quota of women may even be turned on its head in future (Kuhlmann, 2003, 2004). Changing gender relations and new health policies aimed at upgrading general care may intersect and release dynamics into the health system that are hardly predictable.

Physiotherapy: slow advancement of a female professional project

Compared to medicine, physiotherapy is a relatively new health occupation that arrived in Germany at the beginning of the 20th century, and was initially seen as a suitable occupation for daughters from upper-class backgrounds (ZVK, 1993a; Hüter-Becker, 1998). Like other health occupations, physiotherapy was subordinated to the medical profession (ZVK, 1993b), but efforts at professionalisation have been more successful and professional autonomy is higher.

Physiotherapists train for three years in a school-based system, which requires fees and is closely linked to clinical institutions. It concludes with an examination and a state-recognised diploma (Rosenthal and Boxberg, 1997). The Social Code Book V regulates training and the protection of the title 'physiotherapist', but not the control over the occupational field or the market; and as mentioned previously, no register exists for physiotherapists. So far, specialisation has only been formalised in a few areas and has not (yet) led to new professional segments. Functional-technical treatment, mechanical therapies and holistic concepts stand side by side (Hüter-Becker, 1998; Wagner, 1999). At the same time, academic training and new curricula make progress. Several universities of applied sciences have introduced courses of studies leading to a Bachelor degree; some are also beginning to offer Master degrees in order to achieve full access to academic training and titles. There is, however, no career path in Germany that includes medical training, nor are there any lateral connections between physiotherapy and nursing studies.

With respect to the occupational field, the 'employment for upper-class daughters' has developed into an important health care sector that also includes increasing numbers of both self-employed practitioners and men. Physiotherapists make up less than 5% of the health workforce but represent the biggest group of therapists alongside psychotherapists (source: KBV, 2000, p H2). The association estimates a total of 137,000 physiotherapists and a proportion of 20% men. Numbers are on the increase, and nearly half of the physiotherapists work in ambulatory care, with a proportion of 44% practice owners (source: ZVK, 2004, 2005). Data from a regional association of physiotherapy point to shifts within the occupational structure towards self-employment that are correlated to an increase in the quota of men (1993-2003; source: ZVK Bremen, 2003).

A considerable amount of the work of physiotherapists is part of the SHI system and reimbursable CAM prescriptions (Dixon et al, 2003; Scharnetzky et al, 2004), but they also provide numerous services that patients – or customers – pay for out of their own pockets. Most importantly for health policy analysis, SHI expenditure for physiotherapeutic treatment heads the list of complementary therapies; it is five times higher than the occupational therapists in second position (Scharnetzky et al, 2004). It is reported that physiotherapists commonly provide – with or without specialisation – chiropractic and osteopathy, as well as physical therapy that overlaps classical naturopathy (Dixon et al, 2003). Their work thus shows significant overlaps with health care services that are provided by specialists in other countries with their own professional bodies (Saks, 2003b; Kelner et al, 2004).

The employment market shows contradictory tendencies. Negative influences come from the growing numbers of physiotherapists following the creation of many new schools in the 1980s and 1990s (ZVK, 2004); figures given for the 1990s point to a slower but steady increase in numbers (source: KBV, 2000, p H2). In addition, new health policies and significant cuts in SHI care have increased competition for patients. Positive influences, on the other hand, include a continuing fitness boom and demands for preventive treatment and programmes. These new markets promote self-employment and loosen physiotherapy's ties to the medical profession, as patients – or customers – are often not referred by a physician. They also increase the economic leeway and income opportunities, as services are not embedded in the SHI system and patients pay for them out of their own pockets. The growing importance of prevention in health policies might also be a contributory factor in the creation of new markets even within the SHI system. These positive effects on market conditions are furthered by a slight decrease in the number of trainees since 2000 (ZVK, 2004).

It is likely that the changes will lead to yet more differentiation within physiotherapy but not to an overall worsening of market conditions. A previous study supports this assumption: even immediately following the cuts in SHI services in 1996, especially in rehabilitation, the employment market for physiotherapists was judged to be quite good overall. There was still high demand for physiotherapists and job offers in rehabilitation (Kuhlmann et al, 1997).

Positive influences come, above all, from the politics of European integration. In a comparison of European countries Theobald (2004) concludes that the professionalisation of physiotherapy in Germany is linked, in the first instance, to EU politics and only enhanced to a lesser degree by changes in the occupational field. The most serious barrier towards professionalisation is that physiotherapy is not accepted as a profession. Its representatives have only advisory status in the Federal Committee when it comes to negotiations on physiotherapeutic care. The negative impact of this pattern of regulation, which subordinates physiotherapists to the medical profession, stretches far beyond the professional interests of physiotherapists. Even the simple question of 'how many physiotherapists' cannot be answered conclusively.

A major part of the problem is that data on the structure of health occupations is collected by different institutions and according to different classifications (labour market statistics; association of SHI physicians; association of physiotherapists). Indeed, physiotherapy is only sometimes counted as an independent occupation. So the vicious circle continues. Deficits in the macro-political system of corporatist governance lead to deficits in the regulation of physiotherapy and a lack of comprehensive data on which to base decision making.

At present, the quality and efficiency of physiotherapeutic care can hardly be measured. Given these circumstances, decisions on the SHI reimbursement of physiotherapeutic services follow more or less exclusively the interests of the medical profession. The problem is compounded by the fact that research on physiotherapy is in the hands of physicians. Progress in research is slow compared to other European countries (Schämann, 2002), and no specific funding programmes exist for physiotherapy. Interestingly, sickness funds and international organisations support research (Dixon et al, 2003; Scharnetzky et al, 2004), while the government does not take over responsibility of developing databases for evidence-based decision making in physiotherapy.

We are faced with a situation where we can simultaneously observe barriers of corporatist regulation and the advancement of a professional project. Possible reasons for successful professionalisation are therapeutic concepts independent of biomedicine that have managed to forge physiotherapists' own professional identity. In addition, a policy discourse of 'provider cooperation' meets with efforts from within physiotherapy to make use of interdisciplinarity in order to distinguish physiotherapy from other health occupations, especially nursing (Schwewior-Popp, 1994). Furthermore, and equally important, physiotherapeutic services meet with a growing demand from the user (Dixon et al, 2003) and a growing significance in health policy (SVR, 2003; Scharnetzky et al, 2004).

Professionalisation processes provoke different sets of dynamics. The work of physiotherapists and that of physicians and other health occupations overlap in many places, and it can be assumed that competition and conflicts of professional interest will increase. Competition may also derive from the rise of men's quotas and related to this, from changing employment patterns. Similarly to the occupational field, different actors are competing for a 'legitimised voice' in setting the agenda for professional politics. In addition to the association of physiotherapists, other new actors have entered the field of politics, such as academic representatives and a federal network of physiotherapists (ZIPT, 2005).

Taken together, physiotherapy provides a striking example for highly diverse and even contradictory dynamics in health care. While European unification, increasing academic acknowledgement and the growing significance of CAM in health care all further the professional project of physiotherapists, the corporatist order has a countervailing impact. What continue to exist are historically developed barriers and the denial of professional status to physiotherapists, even though new demands on integrated care and more inclusive patterns of coordination run contrary to the established regulatory framework.

Surgery receptionists: limited options for modernising a female occupation

Surgery receptionists are the biggest occupational group in ambulatory care and almost exclusively female (99%). Of all surgery receptionists, 90% work in ambulatory care with a high proportion of part-time workers (sources: Kaukewitsch, 2002; StatBA, 2003b). It is a classic female occupation that has been seemingly untouched by changing gender relations in the labour market and society. We find virtually no self-employment options but full subordination to orthodox medicine and the medical profession. The German term *Arzthelferin* translates literally as 'doctor's helper' and is a clear indication of the subordinate nature of the working relationship and the personal dependency. 'The girls', as physicians often refer to them, have to fulfil a wide range of tasks, mainly defined by what the surgery owner deems suitable for delegation. Their working situation shows interesting similarities with that of secretaries (Savage and Witz, 1992) rather than other health care workers.

A distinct position of surgery receptionist in the health workforce is already laid out in the training system. In contrast to other health care workers, surgery receptionists are aligned to the German 'Dual System' of education. This system comprises three years' practical 'training on the job' and courses at an occupational school, which have low status and no linkage to any kind of higher education. The physician, as the owner of the surgery, is the employer, and representatives of the medical profession are responsible for the organisation and the sitting of the examination. Changes in the curriculum are also defined according to what physicians deem to be necessary in order to fulfil changing tasks in ambulatory care (Richter, 2000).

A further consequence of the Dual System is that surgery receptionists are aligned to the system of occupational representation by trade unions, which collectively negotiate salaries and working conditions. Trade unions, however, are not overly interested in this group because membership is very low. Furthermore, trade unions are not included in the regulatory system of health care. At the same time, surgery receptionists are united in a separate occupational association, together with dentists' and veterinarians' receptionists, which has representatives at the federal and regional levels. This professional body of receptionists is self-regulated but closely related to physicians' chambers and totally excluded from the SHI regulatory system. Thus, two different bodies exist to promote occupational interests but neither has any say when it comes to negotiations on health care. Not surprisingly, the lack of data on surgery receptionists is even greater than in the case of physiotherapists (Kaukewitsch, 2002; StatBA, 2003b).

The labour market for surgery receptionists is inextricably linked to the restructuring of health care and its impact on incomes of physicians: a fall in the latter usually leads to a worsening of the labour market situation for surgery receptionists. This is reflected most clearly in the number of training contracts that are entered into each year and which fell by 7% between 1992 and 2002. The drop is especially visible when we consult the health reform Acts of 1996 and 1997 (source: BdA, 2003). However, unemployment is only half as high (5.3%) and the labour market more stable than in most other segments in Germany, especially those with high quotas of women (Kaukewitsch, 2003). Taken together, the absolute subordination of surgery receptionists to the regime of the medical profession, together with the lack of effective forms of collective representation, lead to negative tendencies in the labour market.

Simultaneously, new possibilities are opening up in the occupational field. The receptionists' association makes use of new demands on surgeries to upgrade the occupational field and promote new career options. For example, on its own initiative a training course for quality management was offered for the first time in 2004, which enables medical and dental receptionists to acquire a formal certificate (ZM, 2004b). However, further options in the wake of new demands on documentation, patient information and prevention are not yet systematically linked to new certificates and specialisation. New chances offered by the market have not, so far, been turned into a strategy to promote the occupational interests of surgery receptionists. The receptionists do not systematically use various new options, opened for instance by the patient information and counselling call centres of SHI funds (Wöllenstein, 2004), to shape a professionalisation strategy. In addition, while changes in the hospital sector provide new employment opportunities, they offer no career tracks for this group (Vogel, 2004). Apart from new opportunities in the workplace, European integration provides a rationale for upgrading qualifications and changing the title of the occupation to 'physicians' assistants' (PAs).

The occupational association employs tactics imported from the professions (BdA, 2003), and calls for new and independent occupational fields, options for self-employment and SHI reimbursement for the service provided by surgery receptionists (BdA, 2003). Although professionalism is gaining ground in the discourse, it does not translate into any substantive change in occupational structure and the system of care. There are no career paths for those who train as surgery receptionists that could lead to other health occupations and professions. New health care requirements have hardly led so far to new formal qualifications of surgery receptionists. They do, however, create new employment possibilities, which may be used individually to improve the employment and working conditions. Simultaneously we observe a significant increase in new employment options and a worsening of working conditions and labour market chances.

Surgery receptionists provide an important resource for modernising the health care system. However, neither physicians nor SHI funds make use of this potential, and health policy totally ignores this occupational group. The significance of surgery receptionists in individual surgeries stands in sharp contrast to the position of this group in the regulatory system. Surgery receptionists are excluded at any meaningful level from the regulatory system and the debates on restructuring of health care. In this situation, conservative forces dominate the field. Paternalism and 'familialism' – the characteristics of the health political culture in Germany (Dent, 2003) – collude to render this occupational group invisible in the corporatist system. Political marginalisation is much stronger than in physiotherapy, and the deficiencies of regulation most obvious. The state does not take over any responsibility for the inclusion of the receptionists in the stakeholder arrangements.

Integrated care: the gap between policy discourse and occupational reality

For over a decade, health policies have attempted to strengthen ambulatory care and improve provider cooperation (Table 3.1). Policy changes have had an effect on the occupational structure if we look at the numbers of physicians. From 1990 to 1999 the proportion of doctors working in ambulatory care rose by 27%, compared to a 14% rise in the hospital sector (source: KBV, 2000, p A3). However, if we look at the greater picture of the total workforce in the health sector, between 1997 and 2000 the ratio of those working in hospitals and those working in ambulatory care was almost turned on its head – although not in the direction that policies intended. The number of those working in hospitals increased significantly (5.4%) but fell in the ambulatory sector (–4.4%). Since 2000 we see an increase in the workforce in ambulatory care and a slower increase in hospitals (source: StatBA, 2003b, p 28). Consequently, the health occupations have not benefited in the same way as physicians from the upgrading of ambulatory care. This general tendency is confirmed with respect to surgery receptionists, as the number of surgery staff fell by around 4% between 1998 and 2002 (source: StatBA, 2003b, p 47). In physiotherapy the picture is more differentiated and points towards an increase of practice owners.

Data do not show whether new policies actually further integrated work patterns. But results clearly highlight that exclusion of these two health occupations from the regulatory framework remains almost unchanged. In this respect a policy discourse of 'integration' and 'coordination' in Germany neither indicates a move towards primary care nor does it substantively alter the corporatist stakeholder arrangement.

Remodelling corporatism from above, from within and from below

The German variety of modernising health care is characterised by a coexistence of innovation and conservatism, depending on the perspective from which we look at modernisation processes. The macro-political scenario of change is characterised by cost containment and marketisation, rolling back the role of the state, the dominance of the key corporatist actors – SHI funds and physicians' associations – and the marginality of user groups and health occupations in the regulatory bodies. Consequently, shifts in the organisational and occupational structure of health care are moderate.

More recently, elements from new governance and a more active role of state regulation are gaining ground and leading to developments that further organisational change, quality management and user involvement. However, a classic strategy of shifting the balance of power towards SHI funds and a focus on control and restructuring of the medical profession linger. A lack of public control of providers and managerial strength of new organisational models remains largely unsolved. The DMPs that are most clearly related to structural change continue to transform corporatist regulation without replacing it. To date, the state has not taken on the task of governing and better coordinating an increasingly hybrid network structure of providers and users that is no longer congruent with public law institutions.

In this situation, new professionalisation projects of the health occupations are establishing themselves alongside the medical profession. But: they do not change the structural dominance of physicians, nor do they systematically link the professionalisation efforts of different occupational groups. At the same time, the medical profession is developing new networks that are not fully under control of the public law institutions; changing gender relations also trigger dynamics that cannot be assessed by looking at institutions and health policy. Furthermore, quality management and performance indicators expand the scope of market logics to the organisation and content of health care, and this, in turn, might promote the interests of some professional groups while weakening others. In addition, the impact of consumer demands may be weak on the institutional level, but these demands feed into an unregulated market, and thereby also enhance changes in the occupational structure.

A new willingness of the government to extend the players involved in regulation challenges the corporatist 'giants' – the SHI funds and physicians' associations – and may pave the way for further changes, such as inclusion of new players from the health occupations. These developments may provoke fissures in the seemingly stable arrangement of physicians and SHI funds. The common diagnosis of 'slow motion' of German corporatism must therefore be reviewed with a critical eye in order to identify more precisely both the drivers and enablers of change, and the barriers towards modernisation. Results highlight that remodelling of corporatism takes places from within, from above and from below. Thus, a more accurate diagnosis is needed of the 'symptoms of old age' of the Bismarckian model and the dynamics of new governance. This is the subject of the next chapter.

FOUR

Drivers and enablers of change: exploring dynamics in Germany

An assessment of international developments in health care highlights significant change on the levels of regulation, organisation and professions that can foster social inclusion. Major elements of global models of modernising health care are taken up in Germany but transformed in a country-specific way. Characteristic of the German model of governance is the centrality of physicians' associations and SHI funds. This polarised model of stakeholder regulation favours the medical profession and nurtures professional strategies of exclusion and hierarchy. The comparative perspective highlights that the most powerful drivers for change, namely a primary care approach and restructuring the organisation of care, comprehensive regulation of all health professions and tighter public control through a system of accountability, are not used effectively in the German system. However, the German health system develops its own dynamics of modernisation and enablers of change. The objective of this chapter is to stake out the social fields of change, the arenas of negotiations and the players involved in Germany. The results of Chapters Two and Three are systematically linked in order to define the drivers for modernisation, and the enablers and switchboards of change, where processes of change cumulate and dynamics can therefore be studied empirically.

German model of modernising health care from a comparative perspective

Modernising health care in Germany is embedded in a global context of changing patterns of regulation and the organisation of providers and changing needs and demands on the provision of care. The transformation covers the organisational and occupational structures as well as the therapeutic concepts of health care; both levels generate clear impulses for change. What is particular to the German system is that marketisation and managerialism are used as a blueprint for restructuring a corporatist system, but not aimed at replacing it. The integration of new regulatory patterns in the existing system is a historically developed model of modernisation in Germany. The coexistence of change and continuity allows for a high flexibility and counts as a source of stability under conditions of economic and social change (Bäringhausen and Sauerborn, 2002). There is probably less uncertainty of the outcome of restructuring in the German system than in market-driven and state-centred systems.

However, the approved balance between innovation and conservation is currently shifting towards a pressure to innovate, and the current pattern of governance encapsulates significant weaknesses. The health system simultaneously faces a number of new challenges from different sides, like increasing economic pressure on the state, new demands in the wake of European unification and globalisation, and new claims on participation from within the classic stakeholder arrangement. New demands are also arising from new players, like consumers and the health occupations, acting from the margins. The merger of global restructuring and local concepts of German corporatism generates its own dynamics, the effects of which cannot be entirely predicted accurately from health policy's incentives and institutional renewal. The emerging dynamics are not only a result of tension between global and national forms of governance. They can also arise from ambivalences and time lapses between structural changes introduced from the top down and models established from the bottom up of the professions. The various regulatory mechanisms and the dynamics and effects on professionalisation and quality of care must be set against the backdrop of reflexivity of social processes and empirically investigated.

The comparative perspective on restructuring highlights the fact that marketisation and tighter bureaucratic regulation are applied simultaneously and professionalism, too, plays an important role in all health systems (Chapter One, this volume). The composition of different regulatory patterns – the market, the state and the professions – is being rearranged. New forms of regulation are emerging that may be described in terms of hybrid network structures of governance. Although the regulatory pattern varies according to national conditions, change in one dimension inevitably provokes change in other patterns. The objective is to assess the emerging new patterns in Germany and their impact on the power structure against the backdrop of both policy and institutional change, and actor-based dimensions of change (Burau, 2005).

Characteristic of the German system is an incremental change and high contingency of medical power due to the complexity of negotiation processes. Consequently, the introduction of elements from new governance does not mean that efforts to preserve the status quo and medical interests are overcome – indeed, under certain conditions competition and 'tribalism' can even be heightened. Networks do not necessarily overturn or replace hierarchy and exclusionary tactics. However, innovative incentives arise from the multiplication of switchboards and arenas for the negotiations of interests. This serves to render the negotiation processes even more complex and the outcome less predictable, which, in turn, generates new and different sets of dynamics. Modernisation processes may increase the risks and uncertainties as to the results of increasing complexity of negotiations. But they may also provide new opportunities for a more inclusive professionalism in a changing health workforce, as well as for the creation of professionals more accountable to the public and defined standards of quality of care (Kuhlmann, 2006a: forthcoming).

The evolving dynamics of primary care (Tovey and Adams, 2001) and changes in the system of health professions and occupations outlined in international studies (Donaldson et al, 1996; Davies, 2003) are clearly more limited in Germany. Nonetheless, the historical monoliths of SHI funds and the medical profession are becoming permeable and more open to new actors. The process of change is not simply slower in Germany but *different* from the Anglo-American countries. This slow pace of change harbours both opportunities and barriers to modernisation. The following sections highlight the drivers and enablers of modernising the German health care system in drawing on the categories outlined in the introduction, namely health policy, especially with respect to quality management and consumerism, the organisation of care and the professions.

Flexibility of corporatist regulation

The complexity of demands on health care calls for the 'remaking of governance' (Newman, 2005a) and mediation between different regulatory mechanisms, actors and interests. These challenges can be answered on the level of institutions; new regulatory bodies and boards of consumer interests and the health professions in the UK are examples of this (Davies et al, 2005; O'Cathain et al, 2005; Allsop and Jones, 2006: forthcoming). The introduction of a Women's Health Advisory Council in the MCO structure in the US (McKinley et al, 2001) is also proof of an increasing significance of negotiations on diverse interests and needs in health care – in this case, gender equality.

Mediation also takes place via informal regulation, thus significantly reducing institutional transaction costs and social conflict. As described in Chapter One (this volume), the medical profession takes over the role of mediator. The key mechanisms are discretionary decision making, public trust in the provision of care and a biomedical knowledge system. The order of professionalism is embedded in institutions and culture, but at the same time, it is socially constructed and open to change. Today's redefined professionalism includes managerial tasks and improved cooperation over the entire spectrum of health professions and occupations. Biomedical care is expanded and complemented by concepts from public health and alternative therapies; lay perspectives are included in the system of health care on micro and macro-levels (see, for instance, BMJ, 2006).

Complex changes on both the levels of institutions and informal regulation impact on the politics and governance of health care in Germany. A global discourse of restructuring is taken up that attempts to strengthen ambulatory care and general practice, prevention and consumer involvement. The strategies of modernisation in Germany, however, focus on two main actors: the provider side is represented by the medical profession and the user side by the SHI funds. This regulatory pattern neglects the conflicts of interests between the professional groups and between SHI funds and the insured. Faced with a scarcity of resources, these conflicts of interests become more important. Although the German welfare system is generally seen as one that embodies complex regulation and multiple steering (Kaufmann, 1997; Rosenbrock and Gerlinger, 2004), in actual fact, the complexity of interests in health care is reduced to two main stakeholders.

Health policy increasingly responds to new demands. New policies aim at user involvement and tighter control of providers. As described in Chapter Three (this volume), these attempts are continuously reinforced with the reform Acts of the 21st century. The crucial point is that the state provides the *framework* for restructuring but does not precisely define *how* new models are to be implemented. Moreover, the state delegates the task of putting policy changes into practice to the SHI funds and physicians' associations. Even within the recently extended regulatory body of the Federal Committee this pattern is not generally changed, although there are now clear signs of state intervention and user involvement.

The legacy of corporatism becomes apparent when we look at recent policy changes that intervene more directly in the joint self-administration and professional self-regulation. The regulatory system and the biomedical approach have both been extended: the negotiations on the first Health Prevention Act in 2005 and the efforts to integrate user representatives into the regulatory bodies, reinforced with the

2004 reform Act, are proof of these changes. Once again, however, the corporatist structure is extended but not replaced by new patterns. This is most evident in the DMPs that aim to shift the balance of power towards the SHI funds. These programmes focus, for the first time, on organisational change and tighter control of the medical profession, but do not significantly alter work arrangements and the dominance of physicians in the system of care.

The state reinforces efforts to engage the SHI funds in its steering goals but not the health occupations; the role of the users of health care services also remains weak and no comprehensive system of accountability and quality management has been established. Health policy's move towards new governance is thus shaped by a classic pattern of corporatist regulation based on two key actors. This marks an important difference to the strategies applied in the Anglo-American countries, where the stakeholder arrangement is increasingly becoming more diverse (Allsop and Jones, 2006: forthcoming). What we must bear in mind here is that regulation of health care is embedded in the German welfare system and therefore difficult to change (Kaufmann, 1997). Characteristic of the system is that new models of health care lead to only weak structural changes and only in certain areas, above all with regard to the arrangement of physicians and SHI funds and in the funding of health care.

The paternalist model of representation of diverse stakeholder interests via physicians and SHI funds is one of the main obstacles to innovation. Most importantly, state regulation is weakest precisely in those areas with the highest levels of dynamics, like the organisation of work and the integration of other health occupations into the system of care. Steering efforts have increased recently but they occur in areas with weaker dynamics, such as bureaucratic regulation and the standardisation of care. Similarly, marketisation and neoliberalism have been expanded in Germany but included in the SHI system. This leads to a reduction of social inequalities caused by market logics in some areas, but, at the same time, weakens the enabling effects of the integration of health occupations and service users. This pattern of governance shapes the options for change and the areas where dynamics can be expected. I will now highlight four conclusions that can be drawn from the situation.

First, weak state regulation and 'controlled marketisation' can be utilised most efficiently by the most powerful actor, in this case the medical profession. Under changing conditions medical power can even be reinforced and re-ensured in ways that run contrary to new policies. The medical profession fills the vacuum left by weak state regulation and makes use of neoliberalism in health care to open up and occupy markets that lie outside the preserve of SHI funding. At the same time, new forms of professional self-regulation and provider organisation are emerging, such as the networks and quality circles of physicians.

Second, by concentrating on the medical profession and macro-politics, the introduced policy changes towards merging of providers and tighter regulation provide most opportunity for the medical profession to control the actual organisation of care. SHI funds do not have the power to directly intervene at the level of organisation, although the options are increasingly expanded. Consequently, restructuring the organisation of care cannot be effectively used as a switchboard for change; and no primary care approach has yet been established. New patterns of organisation of work, such as teamwork and collaboration, are not systematically targeted by health policy and monitored but might emerge from bottom-up initiatives, which, in turn, incite new network structures on the part of physicians.

Third, further consequences result from a regulatory pattern that focuses on physicians' associations and SHI funds. It is not to be expected that the dynamics in the system of health occupations and new professional projects, the success of which can be seen in the Anglo-American health systems (Davies, 2003; Saks, 2003b), will emerge in Germany in the same way. The integration of health occupations is not systematically imposed by health policies. Changes that do come about are rather the result of professionalisation processes and complex changes in the occupational field, including user demands, changing gender relations and European policies.

Finally, concepts of public control and consumers as stakeholders with rights are underdeveloped in Germany and remain marginal even in recent policies that attempt to improve both user participation and quality management. The crucial issue is that regulation is based on the assumption that the joint self-administration of SHI funds and physicians' associations will exercise control of health care. Consequently, no comprehensive 'structure of accountability' is established and policy changes are related mainly to individualised approaches. A global discourse of consumerism in Germany is translated into 'patient-centred care'. Compared with this, an approach based on 'rights' of the users to participate in the health policy process remains weak. For the main part, quality management is reduced to medical care and the physician–patient relationship. In this arena, however, the medical profession is at its strongest and the stakeholder position of users at its most vulnerable. Under these conditions, bottom-up initiatives, such as patient self-help groups, are gaining ground as enablers of change.

While the regulatory pattern of the German health system is becoming more flexible, hybrid forms of governance and informal modes of regulation can be used most effectively by the medical profession. Key areas of change are the network initiatives of physicians and the strategies of quality management.

Consumerism and quality management: the twin strategy of public control

Improved control of providers is a key area of health policy and a driver for modernisation processes. Consumerism and quality management are the favoured strategies. They are two sides of the same coin, and mark a shift from improved technology and physicians' qualification towards managerial and structural change. This shift is summarised as 'scientific-bureaucratic medicine' (Harrison, 1998) and the advancement of 'expert patients' and 'citizen consumers' (Webster, 2002; Clarke et al, 2005). The increasing significance of quality and efficiency calls for new strategies to legitimise professional practice and this, in turn, creates a new arena for negotiations on professional interests. One innovative aspect is that the medical profession takes user interests into account, however limited this inclusion may be in a specific country.

Two basic strategies can be distinguished with regard to user involvement: a market-driven integration in the US, and a state-regulated integration of 'consumers as citizens' in the UK. Notably, the market model of consumerism is complemented by state regulation. This merger of market logic and bureaucracy opens up possibilities to put social differences within the group of users on the agenda; this is most apparent in the US with respect to gender inequality (McKinley et al, 2001). In the Anglo-Saxon model of public participation the user, for the main part, is a non-differentiated actor (Lupton, 1997; Clarke et al, 2005). These findings point to the fact that both market and state regulation provide options to improve user involvement but the effects on quality of care may differ in the various social groups of users. The market-driven health system in the US illustrates the paradoxical situation of the highest level of social inequality coupled with an increasing awareness of gender inequalities and improved monitoring of gender equality in health care.

The differences between the US and the British concepts of consumerism direct attention to the tensions between discourse and structural change, and the significance of regulatory frameworks. With respect to the British system, Newman and Vidler (2006: forthcoming) further outline that even in one country different players use the concept of consumerism in different ways. Furthermore, consumerism plays out differently according to the varieties of welfare state systems. In general, market-driven and tax-financed systems face greater pressure to include the users in the policy process than the corporatist system (Newman and Kuhlmann, 2007: forthcoming). With respect to the latter, a complex network of public law institutions and a health political culture of solidarity acts as a buffer to both diversity of interests and social inequalities. Consequently, the drivers for change are weaker in Germany; this may help to explain the striking deficits in the area of user involvement and quality management (SVR, 2003).

Viewed through the 'German lens', however, the focus on patient-centred care is not only a weakness but also the result of an individualised concept of consumerism, which is based on the freedom to choose a provider rather than on market power and 'control' of providers. Consumerism does not only bring new options for user involvement but also new responsibilities for the government and the corporatist actors, namely SHI funds and physicians' associations.

Health policy takes on the new demands of consumerism. In contrast to the integration of health occupations in the regulatory system, user involvement is increasing. The classic model of representing user rights via the SHI funds, however, has prevented the emergence to any great extent of a comprehensive system of empowering the 'voice' of the user in the health policy process. One consequence is that bottom–up initiatives, from self-help groups of individual patients and independent patient organisations, remain at the margins of the regulatory system. Similar to the integration of health occupations, key conditions of integration are currently not fulfilled in Germany. Service users are not accepted as equal stakeholders and are not prepared for their new role. Furthermore, the dimension of provider *control* and the safety of the public are put on the back burner, and attempts of the state to engage the users in its steering goals are weak. Quality assurance continues to focus on the medical profession and clinical care.

While the strategies of public control are based on national models of citizenship and user participation, quality management of clinical care is highly globalised and standardised. The implementation of evidence-based clinical guidelines and its significance in health care vary from country to country but the legitimatory ground of EBM is similar in all Western states. Evidence-based data are mainly taken from RCTs and many of the studies are carried out in the US; the highest standard of guidelines is negotiated in supranational consensus conferences. Quality management is not only biased towards the body of physicians and orthodox medicine but also towards the social and cultural context of the US and the health care needs of the white – and until recently, male (Healy, 1991) – middle-aged population. We can thus expect global options for more or less similar change in other health systems, and at the same time country-specific limitations of those options.

Overall, the standardisation and monitoring of health care improves the possibilities of integrating new demands and new actors. These options apply to all actors previously excluded from or marginal to the regulatory system. Better control and transparency in health care provide opportunities to define new performance indicators, such as access to health care, gender equality and user satisfaction (Chapter Two). However, one problem with this is that methods, yardsticks and indicators are reduced to biomedical quality standards, despite health policy's attempts to integrate complex conditions of care. This means that what is measured is not what really needs to be evaluated. These deficiencies become ever more apparent and an extension with multidisciplinary methods, including explorative studies and new performance indicators, becomes necessary (Grol et al, 2002; Best and Glik, 2003).

The definitions and measurements of quality do not adequately respond to diversity of health and health care needs. There is an overall lack of standards and data on quality in Germany, but this is especially true, firstly, for the provision of care by health occupations. The data situation is worst for all services not currently included in the SHI system. Secondly, quality standards are related to an illness but not to social differences in the group of users; for example, no advisory groups monitor gender equality. This issue is not or not adequately included in the negotiations on quality of care, although sensitivity is increasingly driven by European gender mainstreaming policies (Kuhlmann and Kolip, 2005).

In conclusion, quality management opens up pathways for change; it promotes the inclusion of new actors and criteria of 'good care'. At the same time, the definition and evaluation of quality and performance indicators remain in the hands of the medical profession. This simultaneously strengthens both the power of the medical profession and that of biomedical indicators and research methods. Further investigations on the inclusion of a wider range of health care demands coupled with the expansion of public control under the umbrella of state-centred initiatives are needed to shift the balance of power. Both are lacking in Germany. At the same time, the medical profession develops its own organisational models of quality improvement and continuous education, like the quality circles.

In Germany, new policies put stronger emphasis on quality management and user participation but both strategies focus on the medical profession and an individualised pattern of consumerism. This reinforces a globalised strategy of quality management that favours the medical profession with a national model of assuring quality via regulation of physicians. Dynamics can be expected within the medical profession but options are reduced for the integration of new actors and approaches in health care as well as public control.

Organisational change: key to restructuring the system of care

Organisational change is one of the most powerful drivers of modernising health care. We must differentiate here between two levels of organisational change: first, the macro-level with the provider organisation, examples of which are the MCOs in the US and the merger of physicians to form PCGs and PCTs in Britain; and second, the introduction of new organisational models aimed at the meso and micro-levels of the provision of care and on changes in the organisation of work. The key strategies here are integrative models of care and the strengthening of primary care.

Organisational development becomes a strategy to catch up with arrears in the modernisation of health systems and to establish new concepts of care. In imitation of reform models introduced in the industrial sector, concepts of teamwork that embody multidisciplinary qualifications, cooperative working arrangements and flat hierarchies are the preferred solution strategy in the health sector. In an NHS Review (NHS CRD, 1999), for example, the obstacles to effective change in health care are identified as high work pressure, lack of communication, insufficient time to carry out tasks, and traditional forms of work; these obstacles are all characteristics involving the organisation of work.

Key conditions of effective integrated caring models are the collaboration of the diverse occupational groups involved, formalised work arrangements, quality management and a cooperative organisational culture. Strong barriers towards integration are medical dominance and 'tribalism' in health care, but also a lack of standards and formalisation of work (Chapter Two, this volume). Taken together these findings point to the fact that state regulation – not merely of the medical profession but of diverse professional groups (Saks, 2003b)

– and jurisdiction of work (Abbott, 1988) are key to the success or failure of new organisational models.

Precisely in these areas, regulation in Germany is weakest and focused on the medical profession (Chapter Three). This is in stark contrast to the global models of restructuring that include a wider range of occupational groups, and govern more directly at the organisational level. In Germany, neither MCOs, like those established in the US (Donaldson et al, 1996), nor a state-regulated merger of physicians, as introduced in Britain (Fulop et al, 2005), are fostered. Although health policy is attempting to shift the balance of power towards the SHI funds, the options are markedly different from those of the managers of the MCOs and within the NHS. SHI funds do not have the power to directly intervene on the organisational level as long as physicians' associations have the monopoly on the provision of ambulatory care.

This powerful position is on the wane, but organisational change remains a result of *negotiations* between SHI funds and physicians; and an outcome of managerial change cannot be taken for granted. Consequently, SHI interventions are generally limited. Furthermore, success in one particular area does not automatically shift the whole system of corporatist regulation. Health policy focuses mainly on financial incentives, while the process of merging providers of health care into networks – and, most recently, medical centres – is currently controlled by the medical profession, and future success of SHI funds is hardly predictable.

Equally important are the differences between global models and German restructuring of the organisation of work. Health policy's attempts to shift the balance of power from in-patient care towards ambulatory care and from specialists to generalists are in line with international developments. Nevertheless, the German version of integrated care differs significantly from the models of primary care developed in Anglo-American health systems. Essential regulatory elements of the latter, such as limited access to specialists and the concomitant gatekeeper function of generalists, have not yet been successfully introduced in Germany. Most importantly, these models are contradictory to the rights of patients to choose a physician, and more generally, to the legal rules and a culture of citizen rights that grant access to an entire spectrum of services covered by SHI care.

Over and above this, new organisational models in Germany continue to focus on the medical profession. They extend the scope of occupational groups involved in a particular area of care – as the DMPs confirm – but they do not significantly alter the dominance of physicians. Most importantly, they do not define *how* the various groups are to cooperate and how to coordinate services. Team-based organisation with fewer hierarchic decision-making and task structures might arise under certain conditions when policies are implemented. But the possibilities of task delegation are neither formally nor legally sufficiently regulated. In this situation, dynamics in the system of care may be furthered, but inclusion of new occupational groups is a matter of ongoing negotiations and the results are not fixed and stable. Similar to macro-level relations between physicians and SHI funds, changes in one area or the success of one occupational group do not necessarily lead to substantive changes in the system of care.

New organisational models in the German health system, especially the DMPs, provide new options for changes in the system of care. At the same time, they are shaped by the deficits of a classic pattern of corporatist regulation that focuses on the medical profession. Under these conditions, options for change in the organisation of work and jurisdiction of that work are more individualised and dependent on organisational context and the specific occupational groups involved in that organisation. Accordingly, we cannot predict whether new policies aimed at organisational change will actually reduce barriers to the integration of the health occupations. We can, however, conclude that the medical profession, in particular, and the success of new professional projects, in general, are important enablers of change.

Shifts in the system of professions

In Anglo-American health systems organisational change has had a significant impact on the transformation of the occupational structure. The strengthening of primary care furthers the upgrading of general medicine, and hereby a professional segment with higher proportions of women. In addition, teamwork and collaboration provide a major source for new professional projects of the health occupations. Of note for the advancement of professionalisation is the fact that the term 'semi-professions' (Etzioni, 1969) is a thing of the past in the Anglo-American debate. Notably, new professional projects are established in a labour market segment with high proportions of women, like nursing and physiotherapy. Improved regulation and increased user demands for CAM, health promotion and prevention may also advance the professionalisation of new groups. Compared to the classical health professions, professional interests of CAM practitioners are more diverse and contradictory and the boundaries more fluid (Saks, 2003b). Similarly, gendering of the actors and projects is more complex.

The chances of integrated care are not effectively taken advantage of in Germany. Health policy has improved the chances, but important conditions are not yet fulfilled. The hegemony of the medical profession and its associations is accompanied by a weak position and a lack of qualification of other health occupations. By comparison with other European countries the education and qualification of nurses and physiotherapists, for example, are not competitive (Krüger, 2001; Theobald, 2004), while surgery receptionists are completely excluded from the regulatory and training systems in health care. The introduction of integrative care and primary care along the lines of Anglo-American models calls for considerable changes at the levels of training and qualification and for new forms to regulate allied health professions and occupations and health support workers.

The lack of comprehensive state regulation and acknowledgement of the health occupations in Germany as professions represents a major obstacle to the realisation of integrated caring models and interprofessional cooperation. Added to this, non-medically trained CAM practitioners are excluded from the SHI system, but doctors – and in part also physiotherapists – increasingly occupy an expanding market for CAM services. The crucial issue is that overlaps between CAM practitioners, the medical profession and other health occupations are not sufficiently regulated by the state but left to market power. Neither qualification and occupational structure nor the regulatory system are transformed in such a way that integrated care can be introduced effectively in Germany.

However, professions do not simply react to health policy; they also enhance change. Progress in the professionalisation of health occupations in Germany is currently under way and changing user demands are opening up new markets for health care services, especially outside the SHI system. In this situation, professionalisation follows pathways that lie outside state protection and state control of the occupational field. A consequence of weak state regulation is that a variety of regulatory mechanisms becomes more important. We can expect dynamics both from the strategies of the medical profession to re-ensure power and control, as well as from new patterns of professionalisation of the health occupations that make use of marketisation and improved formalised qualification, especially against the backdrop of European policies.

Drivers for modernisation and enablers of change in Germany

The comparative perspective highlights the drivers for modernisation that move beyond the rhetoric of marketisation and neoliberalism, and the politics of cost containment. These drivers can be subdivided into those with strong and those with weak dynamics in the system of health care. Stronger dynamics shift the balance of power from the medical profession towards new actors, like the allied health professions, while weaker dynamics enhance change primarily within the medical profession. They may, however, also impact on the system of care but the effects are less clear and more uneven. I would like to recall here the major findings of Chapter Two.

On the macro-level of institutional regulation and occupational structure, the inclusion of the health professions and occupations in the system of stakeholder regulation is a strong driver for change. On the meso-level of health systems the organisation was identified as a switchboard of change, where we can observe the strongest drivers for modernisation, namely primary care and integrated caring models with multidisciplinary qualifications and teamwork approaches. Compared to this, bureaucratic regulation, like quality management and EBM, coupled with the current patterns of user participation enhance weaker dynamics.

Figure 4.1 shows how health policy in Germany applies these drivers. We can observe that all drivers are increasingly applied, and recent policy changes are considerably speeding up the journey (Chapter Three, this volume). In this respect, the German health system mirrors international developments, but the corporatist tradition does not simply give way to global models. Characteristic of health policy in Germany is that it advances the weaker drivers more than the stronger ones. It is interesting to note, however, that in very recent policy changes the tide is turning towards intervention in the organisation of care and thus towards a stronger driver for modernisation. State intervention is not simply strengthened; moreover, the state now acts on a stage that was formerly left to the physicians' associations and SHI funds.

Current developments mark an important shift from classic corporatist regulation with the state acting in the wings towards a new pattern of governance. Attempts to target organisational restructuring are accompanied by interventions in the management of quality and efficiency of care, control of professions and inclusion of users in the policy process that are identified as weaker drivers for change. Not surprisingly, the attempts of the state to apply elements

Figure 4.1: Drivers for modernisation and application to Germany

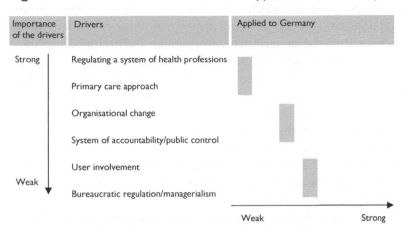

from new governance are shaped by a corporatist tradition and a limited scope of state interventions. The crucial issue, however, is that health policy's move towards stronger drivers for change remains incomplete as it does not include health occupations in the stakeholder system. Nor does it introduce a primary care system or significantly affect the dominance of the medical profession in the system of care. This is not merely a result of a weak role of the state in a corporatist system but a sign of incomplete regulation in an important area of governing health care. Neglecting strong drivers for change on the level of institutional regulation has considerable consequences for modernisation processes on meso and micro-levels: it impacts on the organisation of care and limits the options for change.

The other side of this coin represents new opportunities for the professions to fill in the emerging vacancies in the governing of organisational change and cooperation between providers, and allows those involved to define the indicators and methods of bureaucratic regulation. Owing to the powerful position of physicians and a lack of state support for the health occupations, the medical profession has the strongest resources to successfully use the new opportunities. This is especially visible when it comes to the negotiations with SHI funds on the provision of care, and the definition of standards, performance indicators and the 'evidence' of care. However, the inclusion of the service user brings in a new element of change that challenges all sides – the government, the various professions and the SHI funds. In the same vein, professionalisation processes of the health occupations may also generate their own dynamics that go beyond health policy incentives.

Changes in health policy change the relations between the different players involved in health care in complex ways; under certain conditions even the less powerful players may enhance modernisation processes. Both the lateral initiatives of patients and health occupations, aimed at participation, and those that emerge from the bottom up within the medical profession, aimed at cooperation, have to be taken into account. Although they act from different positions and with different interests and resources, the medical profession, the health occupations and the service users may all pave the way for modernisation processes. Within each of these groups there are 'forerunners' and 'knots' where changes cumulate. Table 4.1 shows the 'enablers' and the main areas where we can expect dynamics in the system of care in Germany.

The networks of physicians, the professionalisation processes of health occupations and the self-help groups of patients can be expected to release dynamics at meso and micro-levels of the health care system. These enablers of change are at the centre of my empirical investigation (research step III). The in-depth study (see the Appendix) shifts the focus from health policy and macro and meso-level regulation towards the meso and micro-levels – the 'switchboards' and 'knots' – of change. It takes on the categories that were previously used to figure out change in different areas in comparative perspective – policy, organisation, occupational structure/professionalisation. However, emphasis is put on actors and agency and processes of change in order to draw a more 'fine-tuned' picture of the dynamics in health care. As described in the Introduction, empirical research takes into account the provider and the user perspective, and different positions in the system of occupational groups with respect to power recourses, gender composition and professionalisation (Chapter Three, this volume).

Table 4.1: Enablers of change and areas of expected dynamics

Enablers	Main areas of expected dynamics
Networks of physicians	Medical profession; organisation of care; SHI regulation
Professional projects of health occupations	Occupational system
Self-help groups of patients	Physician–patient relations; SHI regulation

Part II
Dynamics of new governance in the German health system

The second part of this book highlights the 'meeting' of policies introduced from the top down with the bottom–up initiatives introduced by the professions. It focuses on actor-based changes and the agency of the various players, more related to meso and micro–levels of governance, namely, the new forms of networks and managerialism, new patterns of professionalisation and the impact of the service users (research design step III, see Figure i.1). I ask whether and how the professions take up the key policy issues of modernising health care. Is the German health system giving rise to a new type of a citizen professional, more accountable to patients and the public? Does it promote new patterns of professionalism that better serve the demands of integrated care, quality management and public control of providers? And, concomitantly, does it create a new type of a citizen consumer, one who is fully involved in decision making on health care? The aim of Part II is to highlight the tensions between the innovative and conservative elements of professional self-regulation and corporatism, which release ongoing dynamics in the health workforce and the provider–user relationship. This approach brings into view complex transformations of both governance and professionalism, and the wide room for manoeuvre in the corporatist stakeholder arrangement in Germany.

Part II
Dynamics of new governance in the German health system

FIVE

Hybrid regulation: the rise of networks and managerialism

Changes in the regulation and organisation of work in the German health care system, particularly ambulatory care, are mainly governed by the medical profession. This chapter therefore focuses on office-based physicians and explores how global concepts of managerialism and provider networks play out in Germany. I will assess the developments on the levels of regulation – with respect to professional self-regulation, marketisation and managerialism – and the organisation of work. Analysis of physicians working in networks and gender analysis provide additional information on the enablers of change. Results show that there is no unique voice on regulation but that physicians are creating their own pattern of medical governance. They integrate elements from new governance in order to modernise a conservative system of corporatist regulation without replacing it. This nation-specific pattern of more hybrid regulation does not generate strong dynamics on the macro-levels of institutional regulation and organisation of care; nor does it target the integration of other health occupations. At the same time, regulation and work are shaped by changes that creep into medical work and identities, 'laterally' and from 'below'. Physicians' moves towards cooperation may impact on the structure of health care but in ways that are not fully under the control of the SHI system and not intended by health policy.

Medical network culture and its contribution to modernisation

New health policies attempt to improve the cooperation and coordination of providers in order to overcome the fragmentation of services and better target the provision of health care. Data from my survey reveal that physicians are not generally opposed to new policies, but they see themselves as the 'palace guards' of the health care system. The vast majority, namely 95% to 97%, of the surveyed physicians stated that trust in physicians, high standards of qualification and the robustness of planning of physicians are important conditions for high quality of care. By comparison, the item 'improved qualification and training of health occupations' ranks much lower (80%), and 'improved rights of patient' brings up the tail-light (31%) (ranking: important/less important). There is a clear tendency to incorporate those elements of new policies that do not touch on self-regulation and the interests of physicians. All forms of tighter public control and market regulation are assumed to have a less favourable or even negative impact on health care.

At the same time, the rapid increase of networks and the positive attitudes of physicians on cooperation indicate a *cultural change* in medical practice and identities. Even if one takes into account that data may be biased and attitudes of the total of German physicians less favourable to cooperation, the actual number of members of networks and quality circles is striking. Against the backdrop of a long-standing culture of the office-based physician as an 'autonomous professional' and 'lonely worker' and an occupational structure dominated by solo practices, current changes indicate shifts towards more inclusive patterns of professionalism. Although this marks an important step towards modernising ambulatory care, the networks still lack organisational strength. A representative of an SHI physicians' association compares the networks to a 'meeting of the like-minded', where existing cooperations are further developed and established as formal networks; the boundaries between networks and quality circles are therefore fluid. The innovative aspect of both forms of cooperation is an actor-based change in medical practice that stretches far beyond the institutions and organisations. The following sections will address these issues and outline the tensions and ties that exist between new policies and professional interests.

Coexistence of networks and classic self-regulation

As outlined in Chapter Three, top-down strategies introduced to merge providers into networks have not been crowned with any significant success, while networks and cooperation are springing up within the medical profession. I would like to call to mind the distinction between the networks formally registered by the SHI physicians' associations as provider networks, and all other forms of networks that have either chosen the status of registered charities or do not aim to establish provider networks. Of the physicians surveyed, 29% are members of registered networks and 20% belong to informal networks; a minority of 4% are members of both forms of networks. These findings therefore reveal that 45% of SHI office-based physicians work in networks, a figure that corresponds with the estimates of the surveyed physicians:

44% observed an overall increase in networking and cooperation. Indeed, a smaller study carried out in one of the regions covered by my research found that fully 64% of physicians were members of a network (Nagel, 2004).

At present the phenomenon of the emergence of networks is still confined to the medical profession. Experts from SHI associations confirm that similar developments cannot be observed in other health occupations. Only psychotherapists, who are affiliated to SHI physicians' associations, show an equally high percentage of network members. The lack of networks in health occupations is a reflection of the corporatist structure combined with a health policy that does not stimulate multidisciplinary networks or the merging of health occupations.

The quality circles (*Qualitätszirkel*; see Chapter Three, this volume) of physicians are a further sign of an increase in cooperation within the medical profession. Of the physicians surveyed, 74% are members of quality circles. These groups are part of the system of professional self-regulation and registered by the physicians' chambers. Since the certificate of continuing education required by the 2004 Health Modernisation Act can be earned by credit points for participation in the monthly meetings, membership continues to rise. A survey recently carried out reports quotas of 86% to 90% of physicians who are members of quality circles (Kunstmann and Butzlaff, 2004, p 81), and experts from physicians' associations confirm a rapid increase in the number of quality circles. The quality circles describe themselves as "mini networks" or as "networks of competence", as the interviewed members put it, where cooperation can be learned and quality improved.

Like the networks, the quality circles are a model of bottom-up cooperation with membership open only to physicians. Interviews with group leaders of quality circles, however, reveal that the boundaries are becoming more fluid; for example, members of other health professions and occupations are occasionally invited as speakers. Quality circles thus contribute to the improvement of cooperation with the health occupations, although the organisational model reinforces the division of health care. The crucial point is that the decision on cooperation lies in the hands of the physicians; this issue will be discussed at length in Chapter Six.

The picture of an emerging culture of cooperation is confirmed if we turn our attention to attitudes: 68% of the surveyed physicians perceived cooperation and networking as an important or very important strategy to improve the quality of care. A total of 66% assumed an overall very positive or positive impact on the health care system as a whole. Only 7% expressed negative or very negative attitudes to networks and cooperation (5-point Likert scale). With respect to changes in their own surgery, 51% had improved cooperation with other physicians and a further 27% planned to do so in the near future.

Compared to changes within the medical profession, cooperation with the health occupations is much lower: 19% of the surveyed physicians had introduced cooperation and 22% planned to improve cooperation in their own surgeries. Physiotherapists were more often chosen as partners for cooperation than nurses or social care workers, and cooperation with various health occupations was most frequently stated. Although having a majority of physicians does not further interdisciplinary cooperation, a fair proportion (41%) contributes to the inclusion of the health occupations in the organisation of care. Against the backdrop of the German regulatory system, which excludes the health occupations, actual changes in the surgeries indicate a potential for modernisation that is not stimulated by changing health policies.

The networks and quality circles are a new form of medical self-regulation based on principles of bottom-up and participatory decision making. At present, networks complement – but are not replacing – the classic pattern of institutional regulation via SHI physicians' associations. For example, 67% of the surveyed physicians stated that strengthening the collective representation of physicians has a positive or very positive impact on the health system; only 6% expressed negative or very negative attitudes. The findings indicate that professional institutions do not face an overall loss of significance, but that the terrain is becoming more contested. Although the majority of office-based physicians are not radically opposed to associations, their political power is on the wane. A significant percentage of members do not rely on this traditional form of representation of professional interests. A total of 27% considered that improving the power of associations has no effect on health care. The findings make clear that the medical profession does not speak in unison when it comes to the pattern of professional self-regulation. In this situation, more flexible and hybrid forms of governance are emerging.

Moving beyond the divisional lines of the medical profession

The power structure of SHI physicians' associations is biased towards specialists, men and older physicians. Expert interviews highlight that the relationship between specialists and generalists in the associations is a matter of ongoing conflict within the profession. The power relations have a significant impact on negotiations of global budgets, which have to be distributed among the different professional groups by the SHI physicians' associations. In contrast to this, no consistent pattern of generalists and specialists can be found with respect to membership in registered and informal networks and the quality circles. Similarly, age is not correlated to membership in networks and quality circles. The picture is even more complex when we look at gender relations. Female physicians are marginal in the associations – especially in the higher ranks of SHI physicians' associations – and the neglect of women's interests in professional politics is a matter of ongoing debate (Marburger Bund, 2002; BLK, 2004). However, women's attitudes towards physicians' associations and their membership in networks are similar to that of men.

Analysis of attitudes to associations and networking further highlights the complexity of current transformations in the regulatory structure (regression model: gender, age, generalist/specialist, membership of networks). Membership of a network does not impact on attitudes towards associations; specialised care shows the strongest positive impact ($p<0.000$) followed by female sex and older age ($p<0.05$). With respect to the judgements on networks and cooperation with physicians, younger age ($p<0.01$), female sex and general care ($p<0.05$) correlate with positive statements; not surprisingly, membership of any network has the strongest effect ($p<0.000$). However, the differences in the attitudes to cooperation do not fully correspond to actual change in the surgeries. Here, specialists improved cooperation with other physicians more often than generalists ($p<0.001$); specialists also introduced teamwork approaches in their surgeries more frequently ($p<0.01$).

The findings reveal that specialists and older physicians are more positive in their assessment of powerful associations to serve the demands on health care, while generalists and younger physicians have more positive attitudes to networks. These findings mirror the power structure of SHI physicians' associations. They can thus be explained in terms of interest-based strategies of less powerful players, who are searching for new options to upgrade status and power. The crucial point, however, is that this figure is not entirely congruent with the actual engagement of physicians in networks. Furthermore, women's assessment of the impact of both regulatory models – the networks and the associations – on quality of care is more positive than men's.

The new model of bottom-up professional self-regulation via networks and quality circles crosses the boundaries between generalists and specialists and age groups, as well as the gendered division of labour. The changes may promote less hierarchical relationships within the profession. This is especially visible with regard to members of registered networks: no significant differences can be found for age, sex or specialty. Informal networks show a slightly higher percentage of men ($p<0.05$), and quality circles of generalists ($p<0.001$). Compared with these figures, discrimination is much stronger in classic areas of professional engagement. Specialists ($p<0.000$) and men ($p<0.001$) are more often members of scientific societies; and professional politics is the most biased area, where men ($p<0.000$), older physicians ($p<0.000$) and specialists ($p<0.05$) are in the majority.

The rise of a network culture is observed over the entire range of the profession. Classic forms of regulation and new patterns are not perceived as contradictions, but rather as a form of coexistence. Although network membership does not predict more negative attitudes to the associations, networking is more positively assessed by the less powerful groups in the associations. Interest-related strategies thus play a role in promoting new models of bottom–up self-regulation, and, at the same time, these models do not show a consistent pattern of divisions. Moreover, registered networks tend to equalise the classic divisions of the medical profession. They hereby provide new opportunities for participation of less powerful actors, like generalists and female physicians, and further social inclusion within the profession.

From command and control to commitment: transformation of SHI institutions

The coexistence of networks and associations challenges the corporatist arrangement. It calls for transformations of both physicians' associations and SHI funds. In general, we can observe that changes on the level of SHI institutions lag behind the rapid increase in networks. For example, an Internet search reveals that networks are not top of the agenda for the SHI funds and physicians' associations. Expert interviews with representatives of both sides of the stakeholder arrangement of SHI care confirm this assumption and reveal diverse and even contradictory attitudes to networks. Neither the physicians' associations nor the SHI funds have developed a consistent strategy concerning the inclusion of networks in the regulatory structure. Moreover, we even find a sheer absence of any strategy; for example, a representative of a local SHI fund said that this fund has not discussed the issue, and he is not able to give any statement on cooperation with networks. Nevertheless, what we do find on either side are 'pioneers' of a network policy and a more cooperative regulatory structure.

For example, Germany's biggest SHI fund (AOK) appreciates physicians' networks as 'laboratories of the future', organisations of high strategic value where innovation can be developed and tested under empirical conditions (Schmacke, 2003). Working together with physicians, AOK developed quality indicators of networks (AQUA, 2002). Similarly, the SHI physicians' association of Westphalia-Lippe encourages the merger of physicians into provider networks by offering information and coaching on network management; and the physicians' chamber of Lower Saxony launched a pilot project on quality of care and networking (Stamer, 2002). Moreover, there are voices even from within the physicians' associations that promote multidisciplinary provider networks. We also find the first examples of inclusion of health occupations – for instance, physiotherapists (Weselink, 2004) – in individual contracts between SHI funds and networks. At the same time, more traditional views on the organisation of health care persist.

The findings highlight that the strategies to include new patterns of regulation in the SHI system are not necessarily contradictory between the main corporatist actors but vary within each group. These varieties do not harmonise the differences in terms of interests and power relations between SHI funds and physicians' associations. They do, however, indicate a growing flexibility of stakeholder arrangements and changing constellations of actors in the negotiations on health care. Under these conditions the outcome of negotiations is more uncertain.

We face the paradoxical situation where the corporatist regulatory system allows for high flexibility and increasingly includes new demands on organisational restructuring, but at the same time, this flexibility and the concomitant lack of coordination and organisational strength is a barrier towards modernisation. The crucial point is that neither the SHI funds nor the physicians' associations have the power to actually govern the processes of merging providers (Chapter Three). Although health policy opens the door to selective contracting, and thus undermining the monopoly of physicians' associations on ambulatory care, the SHI funds are not prepared to take over this new role of governing health care. The various SHI funds themselves lack both organisational strength and a comprehensive strategy to merge providers and improve quality and efficiency of care.

Regarding the physicians' associations, current developments do not indicate an attempt to determine the organisational structure of networks, although doctors are often worried about their independence. Even if the associations were to apply tighter rules, the registered networks have several options at hand to undermine these instructions:

"If the SHI physicians' association enters the fray the network can say: 'No, we aren't going to do that, because we don't want to. We'll disband this network'. They can then found a new network with the same members and a modified objective, making a different network. I don't think the association can influence this much. It could, if criteria were defined and it could specifically promote those networks that fulfilled them. That isn't the situation at the moment. It could happen at some point, but it hasn't happened yet." (expert, SHI physicians' association)

In the wake of a rapid increase of networks, the SHI physicians' associations themselves are undergoing organisational change. Some of the associations are introducing new service-centred policies and improving cooperation with the networks. Of the physicians surveyed, 56% welcomed these transformation towards service centres of physicians as a strategy with positive or very positive effects on health care (5-point Likert scale). Notably, membership in a registered network ($p<0.000$) predicts more negative attitudes on the new service policy. This result points to a lack of coordination of the medical profession on different strategies of modernising self-regulation from the bottom up and top down.

Searching for new models of medical governance

The findings highlight that the networks and quality circles do not merely aim at organisational change but at changing the regulation of health care from the bottom up. They thus challenge the traditional pattern of SHI regulation but have not so far developed a clear alternative to the existing model. Interviews with members of quality circles and networks reveal significant criticism of the SHI physicians' associations and physicians' chambers. At the same time, they point to uncertainty about future forms of regulation and highlight a desire to include new models of governing medical care from the bottom up into a classic pattern of institutional self-regulation.

For example, a member of a quality circle of physicians providing general care complained about physicians' associations that do not adequately support the bottom-up initiatives or link these initiatives to the regulatory structure of SHI care. He suggested setting up a new regulatory board comprising the group leaders of quality circles to mediate between the members and the associations. Criticism of physicians' associations was also voiced in the two focus groups:

"We have the bureaucratic types who think they can call the tune [...] but nothing that rocks the boat. Here [in the network] our goal is different; we want to create something where individual physicians feel themselves to be represented by the board, to enter into their wishes and listen to what they think should be represented. I think this is extremely important." (focus group [FG] 1, network, ambulatory care)

The network of women's health care activists described the members of the SHI physicians' associations as "stiff grandfathers", and complained about the dominance of men: "The women working in these groups are often disappointed and quit after a year". This situation seems to be similar in the associations of physicians, psychotherapists and pharmacists. At the same time, the participants in the group discussion point to reasonable changes in the classic SHI institutions. Against the backdrop of increasing political pressure the institutions are becoming more open to innovation and demands from the bottom up. Participants reported for instance that a quality circle of female gynaecologists is increasingly acknowledged by SHI funds and physicians' associations:

"As far as the SHI physicians' association is concerned, it's difficult to be optimistic. But even there something is happening. We have to ask the 'boys' over and say, 'tell us what you think'. And they come. But not without being asked.[...] It's a sort of hybrid form; one in which we are recognised as an informal group, but at least as part of the structure." (FG 2, network, women's health)

The participants emphasised the need for networking and cooperation in order to introduce integrated caring concepts, and to improve the situation of women as professionals and users of health care. They described the building of their own networks outside the established institutions as an important step. However, conditions were now changing, especially with the introduction of a DMP for breast cancer treatment:

"Cooperation is what you might call a legal requirement now. And it's up to us to fill it with content and structure. And that's where it stops being 'our problem'. Now the big ones have to come on board, senior physicians, sickness funds and suchlike. I really think things are changing because there's legal pressure to back it up." (FG 2, network, women's health)

Interestingly, these health care activists judged the changes within the SHI institutions more positively than the provider network of office-based physicians. They observed an "unusual degree of openness" from the SHI funds and physicians' associations. Although they highlighted the necessity of bottom-up networking, they wished for formalisation and inclusion in SHI regulation. It is interesting to note that the physicians working in this multidisciplinary network draw a new picture of partnership with both SHI funds and physicians' association in order to bring the voices of women into the equation. They hereby cross the classic borders of SHI regulation and may contribute to a more collaborative style of negotiations on the provision of health care.

The physicians I studied feel a need to modernise the system of SHI regulation in order to better serve both their own interests and society's demands on health care. However, they are well aware of the privileges of SHI regulation and the uncertainty of all new forms. There is no clear decision on the re-arrangement of medical governance but there is a clear tendency to search for options that transform the existing system of regulation without losing the privileges of state-protected professional self-regulation.

Remodelling professional self-regulation

The rise of a network culture confirms that physicians do not simply react to changing demands on health care but, in a situation where the power of the associations is on the wane, actively create new forms of provider cooperation and coordination of services. This pattern of networks does not significantly change the corporatist principle of professional self-regulation and the hegemonic claims of physicians over the entire field of health care. As the majority of physicians (59%) are not interested in cooperation outside the medical profession we can expect only weak changes in the system of professions and occupations.

However, networks impact sideways on the regulatory structure of SHI care. Physicians' initiatives developed from the bottom up transform the strategies of health policy to merge providers in ways that allow for new forms of professional self-regulation. SHI physicians' associations continue to represent professional interests at the macro-level of regulation, but have lost the power to govern the process of merging and cooperation of providers at the meso and micro-levels; and SHI funds are not able to exercise this role either.

In this situation, the networks and quality circles fill the existing vacuum of governing health care and negotiating professional interests. Physicians claim to be actively involved in regulation, and to transfer the balance of power from the associations towards the members of the profession. Thereby, regulation is becoming more hybrid. These developments provide new options to reduce hierarchy within the medical profession, and may also further a more diverse pattern of negotiations between physicians and SHI funds.

Ambivalence of marketisation and managerialism

Marketisation and managerial tools are generally perceived as powerful strategies to govern medical practice and to reduce professional power. They are key elements of the restructuring of the health care system (Chapter Two, this volume). In terms of classic approaches from the sociology of professions, these strategies act as counter forces to professional self-regulation and lead to deprofessionalisation (Chapter One, this volume). The findings of my survey, however, indicate that marketisation and managerialism impact on professional practice and discretionary decision making in different ways. Tighter control is only one possible effect. At the same time, physicians actively apply these new strategies in order to open up new markets and to reinforce professional power.

If marketisation is related to patients, the majority of the surveyed physicians (82%) judged co-payment as a positive or very positive strategy to improve health care (82%). In line with this approach, they extended 'tailored services' (Table 3.1, Chapter Three) or planned to do so in near future (64%). Data indicate that the majority of physicians undermine the cultural value of solidarity of the SHI system in order to increase individual financial benefit. This is especially visible in the group of specialists, who have better opportunities than generalists to expand tailored services. Although attitudes to co-payment of patients were similar in both groups of office-based physicians, specialists introduced tailored services more often than generalists in their surgeries ($p<0.000$). Furthermore, women's attitudes on co-payment of patients were slightly more negative than men's attitudes ($p<0.05$), but the statements on actual changes in their own surgery do not reveal any significant gender difference.

Economic logic not only invades the physician–patient relationship but is more generally applied to medical practice. The findings from the survey highlight that professional attitudes are malleable according to new policies and changing conditions of health care; the majority acknowledged accountability to financial conditions of health care. A total of 61% stated that 'improved cost consciousness' of physicians is an important condition of high-quality care (ranking: important/less important). Although physicians are increasingly willing to take financial aspects into consideration, major controversy remains on how to improve efficiency in the health care system. This is especially visible if we look at the most contested area, namely, the monopoly of SHI physicians' associations on contracting (Chapter Three, this volume). The attitudes of the majority of physicians were in line with the traditional politics of the associations: 81% expected a negative or very negative impact on health care from individual contracts with SHI funds (5-point Likert scale). With respect to the attitudes on MCOs, the statements were more heterogeneous. About one third of the physicians expected a negative or very negative effect, but 22% a positive or very positive impact on health care (5-point Likert scale).

Although the majority had traditional attitudes on contracting, 10% to 18% of the surveyed physicians explicitly welcomed competition and flexibility of contracting. In addition, about 10% did not expect any effect on health care from changes in contracting and 42% expected none from MCOs. Set against the high relevance of collective contracting as the 'core' of corporatist regulation and professional power, these findings point to significant fissures in the homogeneity of the medical profession. Physicians no longer stand united against flexible contracting and MCOs; neither are attitudes unanimous on the other side. Similar to the attitudes on new patterns of professional self-regulation, no new model of contracting that could replace the key role of SHI physicians' associations is on the horizon.

Physicians are not willing to accept a mere shift in responsibility for ambulatory care from the physicians' associations towards the SHI funds but are searching for new options. Compared to market-regulated contracts, the attitudes on state-centred and managerial patterns of regulation were slightly more positive and diverse, although the majority was opposed to global budgets (71%). The attitudes of physicians point to a desire for new models of organising SHI care, that provide better opportunities for individual action without losing the benefits of collective market power in the negotiations with SHI funds. Thus, attitudes on new models of provider regulation may be explained in terms of interest-related strategies. Not surprisingly, this is especially visible when we look at the attitudes towards the gatekeeper function of generalists: 79% of providers of general care, but only 13% of the specialists expected a positive or very positive impact from a gatekeeper model (5-point Likert scale). Differences between generalists and specialists diminished with regard to attitudes on contracting, managed care and global budgets.

With respect to the enablers of new patterns of SHI regulation, analysis shows no consistent relation between the power structure of the medical profession – age, gender, specialty – and attitudes on new regulatory models – individual contracting, global budgets, MCOs. But specialists and older physicians are more willing to change classic SHI regulation. Accordingly, the most powerful groups within the profession do not act as conservative forces but as forces for change. Gender does not significantly impact on the attitudes on SHI provider organisations. Additional information from female office-based physicians highlights that women do not expect new regulatory models per se to promote gender equality, but each model has its specific options and problems for women in the profession. Similar to the networks that cross the classic lines of divisions within the profession, the changes in the organisation of SHI care may further a re-division of the medical profession. There are no signs, however, that a move towards market-based regulation of SHI care stimulated by health policy actually reduces hierarchy within the profession. Moreover, the powerful players are more in favour of these policy incentives.

Tension between policy incentives and individual motives for change

Health policy is mainly driven by economic logic, and incentives for change are based on the assumption that physicians also act according to this logic. In contrast to this assumption, professional practice is shaped by a number of different motives and demands (Nagel, 2004; Chapter Three, this volume). The following section addresses the question as to whether and how network membership and attitudes on new regulatory models are linked to the economic situation of physicians. This relationship is assessed for two items that are usually used as rough estimates of physicians' income: the 'quota of privately insured patients' and the 'number of SHI certificates per patient per quarter' (*Krankenscheine*).

The latter indicator is specific to the German health system and needs some explanation. SHI patients formerly received a certificate from their sickness fund that covered all necessary health care and all visits to the doctor for a period of three months. In the case of illness the first doctor they consulted – whether a specialist or generalist – received the certificate and sent it to the SHI fund, which then reimbursed the patient for all treatments. In the case of consultation of other doctors, patients needed a further certificate from the first doctor but were also able to request a second certificate from the SHI fund. This model of reimbursement of medical care has been modernised with the introduction of patient chip cards, and since the 2004 Health Modernisation Act, 'doctor hopping' and specialised care are to be reduced by an out-of-pocket fee for consultations without referral by a generalist. However, the basic principles of reimbursement, at present, remain unchanged. Higher numbers of SHI certificates and privately insured patients thus predict a higher income, although these indicators do not reveal actual earnings. In addition, individual estimations on the financial development in their own surgeries are taken into consideration as an impacting factor, and the item 'working hours' is added to the multiple regression model described in the previous section.

The findings reveal highly complex relationships between new regulatory models, individual perceptions and the financial situation of a surgery. Most importantly, however, network membership does not impact on the individual judgements regarding a surgery's financial prospects, and the statistical indicators of the economic position do not show a consistent pattern. Compared with physicians who do not belong to a network, we notice a lower quota of privately insured patients and a higher number of SHI certificates for members of registered networks. Informal networking is correlated to higher numbers of privately insured patients, and thus points squarely in the opposite direction. Gender is not correlated to individual perceptions nor to the quota of privately insured patients, but women have fewer SHI certificates than men. Compared with that of men, the financial situation of female physicians seems to be slightly more negative. With respect to differences between generalists and specialists, the indicators used here point to lower incomes of generalists, and thus confirm the picture drawn from official statistics (Chapter Three, this volume). At the same time, generalists expected more positive developments of the financial situation than specialists. This difference may be a reflection of new health policies that attempt to upgrade general care.

Data highlight that the move towards cooperation and networking is not governed by promises of financial benefits. At the same time, interest-related strategies provide some explanations for the attitudes on new regulatory models. Higher numbers of privately insured patients predict more positive attitudes on marketisation and competition. With respect to managerialism, however, only positive expectations on their own financial perspective predict more positive attitudes. Furthermore, indicators of the financial situation are linked to membership in a network but in different ways. The findings make it apparent that new provider models and the rise of a network culture are nurtured by a wide range of professional interests that may even be contradictory.

In addition, physicians present themselves as acting in accordance with professionalism and altruistic values rather than economic logic. For example, 'satisfaction of patients' (65%), 'self-determined work' (62%) and 'reduced workload' (45%) were stronger motives for change in their own surgery than financial gain (37%; ranking 'very important' on a 3-point scale). These figures point to a gap between health policies that attempt to stimulate change through financial benefits and the attitudes and wishes of physicians. This gap provides some explanations for the failure of the pilot projects introduced by the 2000 Health Care Act (Chapter Three, this volume) that were based on economic incentives for change.

The findings confirm that interest-related strategies driven by financial motives stand side by side with professional values of 'autonomy' and altruistic logic. We can conclude from these results that professionalism does not stand as a 'third logic' (Freidson, 2001) or a wall against marketisation and managerialism. Moreover, it plays host to very diverse strategies to promote professional interests. Diversity of interests and professional values lead to multiple areas of change, thus rendering the enhanced dynamics highly complex. Network membership does not significantly impact on attitudes towards new models of provider regulation; interest-related strategies provide some explanations but do not show a consistent pattern. Neither health policies attempting to upgrade general care nor the increase in female physicians point to a consistent pattern of change in the regulatory system of SHI care. The complex relationship between policy changes and changes within the medical profession will be further outlined with respect to regulatory tools more related to the micro-level of health care.

Linking quality management and public control to professional interests

The growing demands on quality management and control of providers directly impact on professional practice. In this arena both the conservative forces and the capacity of professionalism to assimilate new demands are most apparent. Attitudes on the major goals of health policy to control medical practice (5-point Likert scale) show the following picture: 68% had a positive or very positive attitude to 'binding quality standards'. Regarding the item 'legal obligations of continuing education', however, the figure fell to 32%, and 'certification of surgeries according to ISO norm' – a standardised measurement developed in the industrial sector – ranked even lower (27%). Notably, nearly a third of the physicians surveyed expected negative or very negative effects on health care from these two strategies. Results indicate that about one third of physicians are in favour of new health policies, and the majority can be expected to be actively or passively opposed to public control. This figure corresponds to an even higher percentage (83%) that did not expect improved patient rights to have any positive effect on health care.

Attitudes towards tighter control of providers are further analysed with respect to age, sex, specialty and network membership (regression model). Results highlight that networks do not impact significantly on physicians' attitudes to public control. The only exception to this is informal networking, which predicts more positive attitudes on 'legally binding quality standards' ($p<0.01$). Female sex is a strong predictor of more favourable attitudes for three of the four items, while age and specialty do not show the same strength and consistent pattern.

In contrast to attitudes related to tighter control, at a first glance physicians' statements on improved quality management are more homogeneous and in line with health policy. Regarding the different tools to improve quality, the 'quality circles of physicians' rank first (79%), followed by 'second opinion' (75%), 'guidelines' (74%), 'evidence-based medicine' (72%), and 'networking and cooperation' (66%). Furthermore, 53% of the physicians stated that they had introduced strategies to improve quality of care in their own surgeries and a further 27% said they planned to do so. With respect to differences within the profession, the female sex shows the strongest correlation with positive attitudes on quality management, and younger age also predicts more positive attitudes (regression model: age, sex, generalist/specialist, network membership).

A gendered pattern of quality management is not confirmed when we look at the actual introduction in physicians' own surgeries. Here, membership of a network is the strongest predictor for quality management. Although not with the same strength, it also predicts more positive attitudes on guidelines, EBM and quality standards compared to the group without any network. The results correspond to the Health Monitor Survey that compared office-based physicians in solo and group practices: here, working in group practice was related to more positive attitudes on quality management (Kunstmann and Butzlaff, 2004). Data from my survey reveal that networks are enablers of quality management but they do not further public control to any significant extent; I will return to this issue in the next chapter.

Physicians are not opposed to regulation and control in general. They are willing to improve quality of care and investigate continuing education. An average of three quarters of physicians in the survey welcomed the new managerial tools and established quality management in their own surgeries. The high quotas of members of quality circles (74%) and scientific societies (78%) are also proof of this willingness. In addition, the Health Monitor Survey demonstrates that 55% of office-based physicians used clinical guidelines in their own surgery and about 80% expressed positive attitudes to EBM (Kunstmann and Butzlaff, 2004). Accordingly, physicians do not necessarily perceive managerialism and bureaucratic regulation as a threat to professional autonomy and discretionary decision making. Moreover, new health policies and new managerial tools may intersect with professional interests in positive ways (see Chapter Six for further discussion). The crucial point is the hegemonic claim of physicians on the measurements and standards of quality of care, and the strategies to improve it. There is a clear tendency to be more in favour of regulatory tools that are firmly in the hands of the medical profession.

Gap between cultural and organisational change

The rise of networks and more positive attitudes on cooperation do not fit easily into the occupational structure of ambulatory care in Germany. As described earlier in Chapter Three, individual practices make up the majority, although the number of group practices is slowly increasing. Material from the survey further reveals that in most group practices two physicians work in partnership (70%); surgeries with more than four partners are the exception; the average number of staff (including surgery receptionists) is six per surgery. Accordingly, the overall positive attitudes on cooperation do not significantly accelerate the organisational merger of physicians. The individual surgery, even if it is organised in partnership, remains the dominant organisational unit of ambulatory care. The following section takes a look at the changes in this organisational unit.

Continuity of classic work arrangements

Long working hours and frequent patient contacts are a characteristic work pattern of office-based physicians in Germany. On average, physicians in my survey worked 54 hours per week; they had frequent patient contacts (58 per day) and no working day reserved for commitments other than the treatment of patients (82%). Part-time work plays no significant role for office-based physicians. If part-time is defined according to the common pattern of 20 hours per week in Germany, only 0.5% of all surveyed physicians choose this model. Even more surprisingly, only 7% fit Germany's regular work pattern of a 38.5-hour week, while the vast majority (93%) worked longer hours. Asked about the hours they would ideally wish to work, the average of 41 hours comes closer to the regular work pattern, but only 2% wished for a 20-hour working week. Unsurprisingly, complaints of a high workload were the rule, and occupational satisfaction was low.

Physicians perceived the current trends in their own surgeries as negative or very negative regarding workload (59%), occupational satisfaction (63%) and future prospects (76%) (5-point Likert scale); the majority even expected an increase in their 'bureaucratic' workload. Specialists and men perceived their occupational perspective as more negative than generalists and women; and the older physicians in my study expressed more pessimism with regard to workload and occupational satisfaction (regression model: age, sex, specialist/ generalist, network membership, working hours). Surprisingly, women were more optimistic than men regarding their individual situations, although statistical data and research on career progress point exactly in the opposite direction (BLK, 2004; Blättel-Mink and Kramer, 2006: forthcoming).

Membership of a network does not significantly impact on any of the items related to the individual situation, but higher working hours are correlated to negative perceptions of occupational workload, satisfaction and perspective. Taken together, physicians seem to be a highly pessimistic and dissatisfied professional group. Given that the satisfaction of providers has positive effects on quality of care (Leiter et al, 1998), and a high frequency of patients undermines patient-centred care, the pessimistic stance of office-based physicians is a serious risk to the quality of care. Notably, an increase in networks does not improve the situation.

Although high workloads and dissatisfaction are general phenomena in the medical profession, gender differences are striking. Female physicians are markedly different from their male colleagues with respect to working hours. On average, women with children worked six hours fewer per week than men with children. This difference is in part related to the gendered pattern of childcare but even in the group without children women worked two hours less than men ($p<0.05$) (multiple regression: age, sex, generalist/specialist, women/men with children). This means that motherhood does not provide a full explanation for the gendered pattern of working hours. This is even more obvious when we look at the wished-for ideal: on average, women wished to work four hours less than men ($p<0.000$), and children have no significant impact on this finding.

Gender differences persist if we look at the work arrangements. Female physicians more often had working days without patient contacts ($p<0.001$), and treated six patients fewer per day than men ($p<0.000$) (regression model: age, sex, generalist/specialist, network membership, working hours). The gendered pattern of work is striking but female physicians, even those with children, do not fit the common pattern of women's labour market participation in the western part of Germany. Women's occupational breaks are more frequent and longer than in the group of male physicians, but lower and shorter compared to other occupational fields in Germany (Bird and Gottschall, 2004). Furthermore, the average working hours of female physicians are even higher than in the population at large. Accordingly, the continuous increase in female physicians (Chapter Three) enhances shifts in the work pattern but does not significantly alter the dominant model of continuous employment and long working hours, which is characteristic of a 'male' pattern of work.

Apart from gender, specialty and network membership also impact on work arrangements. Generalists treated five patients per day more than specialists ($p<0.000$). Members of registered networks also had a significantly higher frequency of patients per day, and membership of any network predicts longer working hours (regression model: age, sex, generalist/specialist, network membership, working hours). Accordingly, an increase in networks reinforces a traditional pattern of medical work characterised by long working hours and frequent patient contacts, and thus reinforces pessimistic perceptions of the individual situation and occupational prospect. Overall, the dynamics strengthened by networks point exactly in the opposite direction of those arising from the growing quotas of female physicians. Different sets of dynamics may thus be neutralised when it comes to changes in the work pattern.

Innovating surgery management

Signs of organisational change appear if we look at the management of the surgery. Most importantly, 71% had introduced teamwork and 15% planned to do so in the near future. These statements correspond to data on the organisation of work: 69% said they have regular team meetings, 5% of which had less than one meeting per month; 54% had one and 21% two meetings per month, and 21% met at least once a week. The strategies to improve quality management described in the previous section are a further sign of transformations in the surgeries. This picture is reflected in surgery management; 50% had already improved and 36% planned to improve the managerial style. In addition, about half of the surveyed physicians had introduced more flexible surgery opening hours. With respect to changes in the physician–patient relationship, 64% had improved patient information (24% planned), and 58% partnership with patients (20% planned). Similar findings of 60% to 70% positive attitudes on items related to well-informed patients are reported from the Health Monitor Survey (Kunstmann and Butzlaff, 2004).

The findings indicate that approximately 80% to 90% of office-based physicians are willing to improve surgery management. Some of the strategies explored, such as 'global' models of restructuring (Chapter Two, this volume) are applied in German surgeries, but others remain weak. This is especially true for cooperation with the health occupations: as described previously, only 19% had improved cooperation, and no group of physicians can be identified as enablers of inclusion of the health occupations in the system of care. Set against the much higher percentage of teamwork approaches in the surgery, the findings point to contradictions and tensions between physicians' definition of teamwork and the inclusion of health occupations. I will come back to this issue in Chapter Six.

The picture of an innovating profession that furthers restructuring from the bottom up without significant transformations in the system of care will be further analysed with respect to change agents. The following three groups can be expected to enhance dynamics: networks and generalists, as those groups favoured by health policy, and women, who are making inroads into all areas of the profession and may also be encouraged by society's growing sensitivity with regard to gender inequality. I will analyse the interplay of different actor-based changes with regard to the main indicators for innovation: improved cooperation with physicians, team approaches and team meetings in the surgery, improved management of the surgery, quality management, extension of tailored services, improved patient information and partnership with patients, and networking with health occupations (regression model, age, sex, specialist/generalist, network membership).

Membership of any kind of network is a predictor for teamwork and improved management ($p<0.01$), and cooperation with health occupations ($p<0.000$); informal networks also impact positively on patient information and partnership with patients ($p<0.001$). Gender shows no significant effects on surgery innovation with the exception of higher quotas of women than men, who improved patient information ($p<0.05$) and partnership with patients ($p<0.001$). Specialists introduced almost all strategies more often than generalists, but cooperation with health occupations is not related to specialty, age or gender. This is surprising, as female sex and general care predict slightly more positive judgements on improved training of health occupations as an important condition of high quality of care ($p<0.05$; ranking: important/less important). Obviously, these attitudes did not translate into frontline changes in their own surgery.

In conclusion, physicians' move towards networking and cooperation is accompanied by organisational change within the surgeries. Network members and specialists promote innovation of surgery management, and networks also contribute to teamwork approaches and cooperation with health occupations. However, changes do not touch significantly on the organisational structure of health care and the work pattern of office-based physicians. We can observe a gap between cultural and organisational change that is likely to release ongoing dynamics in the system of health care.

Dynamics of networks and shifting gender composition

The findings indicate that dynamics are provoked by different players and drivers for change, and may thus play out differently in the various arenas of health care. This section therefore assesses the interplay of different 'sets of dynamics'. With respect to the institutional framework the emerging system of network governance from the bottom up of the profession challenges all players in the corporatist system, but a clear direction of change in the power structure both of the stakeholder arrangement and within the medical profession cannot be identified.

Furthermore, changes in the key principles and values of the SHI system – collective contracting, reimbursement and full coverage of health care services – are not driven by networks, but by the interest-related strategies of physicians. This is especially true for the most powerful group, the office-based specialists. Consequently, dynamics provoked by marketisation and competition – the strongest policy incentives – may run contrary to the attempts of upgrading general care; tensions are thus embedded in health policy itself. Not surprisingly, we do not find any significant proof that an upgrading of general care would provoke stronger dynamics or a consistent pattern of change in the health system – this finding corresponds to the picture drawn from statistics (Chapter Three). A lack of any consistent pattern of change is also true if we look at demographic change in the medical profession. We do, however, find a number of weaker dynamics that point towards uneven changes emanating from both demographic change and polity shifts towards strengthening general care.

With respect to meso and micro-level regulation of medical practice, networks promote the improvement of quality management but not of public control, while increasing numbers of female physicians impact positively on both levels. As far as work patterns are concerned, networks cannot be expected to enhance dynamics in any significant measure. An increase in female physicians predicts change in the working patterns but does not significantly change the management of surgeries or promote innovation. In this area networks are the 'change agents'; they touch on the organisation of work and the system of care, and may thus enhance dynamics in an area that has been identified as a switchboard of change (Chapter Four).

However, the image of networks as 'change agents' crumbles when we look at the expert–patient relationship and the content of care; changes in these areas were also identified as predictors of dynamics (Chapter Four). Membership in a network shows no significant effect on any of the attitudes related to patient rights and health prevention, but increasing quotas of female physicians promote change (regression model: age, sex, generalist/specialist, network membership). Female physicians ranked 'patient rights' more often as important conditions of high quality of care than men ($p<0.000$); younger age and specialised care were also weaker predictors of positive attitudes ($p<0.01$) (ranking: important/less important). However, when asked for a statement on improved patient rights, only the female sex predicts more positive attitudes ($p<0.000$) (5-point Likert scale). Women physicians – and generalists, too – also expressed more positive attitudes on improving health prevention ($p<0.000$) (5-point Likert scale).

The findings indicate that increasing numbers of female physicians have a stronger positive impact on social inclusion of patients, public control and the inclusion of preventive care in orthodox medicine than any changes in the composition of age or provider arrangements.

Accordingly, shifts in the gender composition enhance dynamics in the areas not touched on by networks. And in turn, networks enhance dynamics in the regulatory framework and the micro-level of organisation, where changing gender composition does not have a substantial impact.

Towards a new medical governance

Results show that the German health care system faces significant transformations towards modernisation that are driven by changes within the medical profession. Office-based physicians actively take part in the making of a new medical governance. This pattern embodies both a potential for modernisation and conservative forces. Physicians increasingly apply elements from new governance and open coordination in order to modernise self-regulation. They hereby counteract health policies that attempt to shift the balance of power towards the SHI funds, with the search for an alternative to the classic corporatist arrangement, however tentative and incomplete this alternative is at present. A characteristic feature of developments in Germany's health system is that of different areas of change and various enablers. Changes occur on meso and micro-levels of health care, and do not easily translate into institutional change. Consequently, changes cannot be grasped in terms of institutional regulation and structural change. Rather than a simple decorporatisation – or decline of medical power – we face a complex transformation of both corporatism and professional self-regulation from inside the profession.

An increase in networks and cooperation is, first and foremost, an indicator of cultural change that covers all groups of office-based physicians but does not march in step with structural change. However, in terms of new institutionalism the emerging network culture impacts in complex ways on the 'institutional environments' in health care. This impact and its dynamics become visible when we compare network members to those without any professional network. As described in the previous sections, networks have the capacity to advance modernisation processes in some areas of regulation and organisation of health care, while change in the expert–lay division can be expected from an increase in female physicians. These examples highlight a potential for modernising health care emanating from within the medical profession.

When it comes to public control and substantive change of the organisation of providers, however, conservative forces enter the picture. Medical power continues to exist in a more flexible and 'timely' version.

While creating a citizen professional, who is more willing to accept accountability and to apply managerial tools, the medical profession elegantly succeeds in bypassing calls for public control and organisational change. This model of medical governance overlaps with health policy that calls for a citizen professional more accountable, first and foremost, to the politics of cost containment, but it does not advance comprehensive organisational restructuring and public control. Conservatism of the medical profession is thus nurtured by health policy and the corporatist arrangement. At the same time, signs of more inclusive patterns of regulation and organisation of care are emerging from both changing policies and changes in the medical profession.

The transformation of the German health system is a very slow process indeed, but a move towards incremental modernisation is taking place. Changes are embedded in organisational contexts and professional self-regulation. The corporatist pattern of modernisation may thus promote more sustainable change than state-regulated or market-driven systems. An innovative potential of bottom–up modernisation is particularly manifest when we look at the 'enablers' in the medical profession. In the long run, the growth of networks and the increase in the number of female physicians may boost developments towards modernisation in those areas that predict stronger dynamics and that are not adequately stimulated by health policy. However, the different sets of dynamics may also play out in unintended ways, thereby releasing new uncertainties in the governance of health care. They simultaneously provide new options for and limits to the 'remaking of governance' (Newman, 2005b) that are further explored in the next chapter.

SIX

Transformations of professionalism: permeable boundaries in a contested terrain

Professionalism is increasingly applied to the entire field of health occupations and falling into a more flexible and contextualised regulatory order pattern, which different actors can make use of in various ways. This chapter will explore the varieties of and opportunities for a more inclusive professionalism. I will assess changes in three occupational groups that act from very different positions in the health care system and set the dynamics against new demands on health care and citizenship. The findings highlight the flexibility and power of professionalism to transform itself. Physicians develop new strategies that link professionalisation to elements of new governance; physiotherapists expand marketisation, improve academic training and bypass the control of physicians; surgery receptionists refer to professionalism, despite a lack of resources and a gender identity that clashes head on with professionalisation. An increasing diversity provides new opportunities for the softening of professional boundaries. However, interprofessional dynamics remain weak and medical power strong, as the state fails to set up structures that better coordinate the entire workforce. The options of an emerging inclusive professionalism do not, therefore, translate easily into a collaborative health workforce and 'citizen professionals' that better serve public demands on health care.

Medical profession: linking professionalism and new governance

Medical practice is challenged by the logics of marketisation and managerialism, and by claims for accountability and the participation of new actors in health care. These challenges are under the spotlight of public discourse and research on the medical profession. However, pressure 'from outside' is only one side of the coin, and this perspective nurtures the assumption that professionalism is threatened by new health policies. In reality, we find new demands 'from within' the profession. We have learned from the results of the survey that physicians claim more active participation in professional self-regulation and are searching for new forms of cooperation.

It is precisely this perspective that underlines the fact that professions are part of changing modes of citizenship as a super structure of modernisation (Chapter One, this volume). Accordingly, transformations of professionalism must be assessed as reflexive processes (Giddens et al, 1994) provoked on different levels and nurtured by different and even contradictory interests. Developments can be explained in terms of changing interest-based strategies of the medical profession related to changing health policies and new demands on health care. Three dimensions of transformation will be assessed: marketisation, managerialism and networking.

In their unadulterated versions, marketisation and managerialism – the strongest policy incentives for change – do not appeal to professionalism and, unsurprisingly, are not welcomed by the majority of physicians (Chapter Five, this volume). However, market logic and managerialism are not 'aliens' invading the terrain of health care with a view to conquering the professions. Moreover, these regulatory models have several links to other tactics familiar to professional projects, which provide bridges for inclusion in professional strategies and order patterns; the struggle for market power, in particular, is a classic element of successful professionalisation (Larson, 1977).

In a situation where state protection and the collective power of the associations are on the wane and a scarcity of resources reinforces competition within the profession, the struggle for market power takes on a new meaning: individualised tactics and more flexible strategies to defend professional status are gaining ground. Interest-based strategies are not detached but becoming more independent of both state protection and corporatist power. Increasing user power and the exclusion of various services from the SHI system – another side of the individualisation of health care – contribute to these developments.

As described in Chapter Five, physicians respond to marketisation and competition with a double-edged strategy to uphold their professional interests. They are searching for new patterns of professionalisation that ensure both collective action under conditions of increasing competition and greater room for manoeuvre for individual action. This search creates new demands on more flexible and less hierarchical regulation, and calls for a better coordination of the diversity of interests within the medical profession. Subsequently, it points to the options provided by 'new governance' as a changing mode of organising complex stakeholder relations and the diversity of interests in the public service sector. As we shall see, physicians are 'conquering' the innovative potential of new governance as a tool for modernising professionalism 'from within', thus counteracting health policy attempts to reduce medical power.

Interest-based strategies in transition: towards network governance and managerialism

Networking and managerialism play a crucial role in the transformation of a historically developed 'gaze' of the medical profession – based on exclusion and hierarchy – into a 21st-century health care service, which is more open to participation of both the professionals and the service users. Networking is not merely an organisational strategy to merge providers and remodel self-regulation but a highly complex new pattern of professionalisation based on managerialism, cooperation and participation, and the decentralisation of power. Physicians are capable of selecting precisely those elements of new governance that allow for transformations according to professional interests.

Transformations are most obvious in the area of quality management. Survey data indicate that physicians welcome and apply tools from managerial regulation in order to improve quality assurance and the management of the surgery, while all tools related to tighter public control are assessed more negatively (Chapter Five). Interview material further highlights the tensions and ties between managerial tools and professional interests. For example, the certification of surgeries according to ISO (International Organization for Standardization) standards (developed in the industrial sector) was described as a mere technical strategy, "that is a contradiction to our approach of collegiality, confidentiality and trust [...] and, in some respect, it puts us in chains" (FG 1, network, ambulatory care). Similarly, a member of a quality circle characterised the continuing education of physicians as "important, but any kind of control and force are nonsense". Several participants emphasised the power of physicians to bypass and outflank all strategies aimed at the tighter control of the quality of care and the qualification of doctors.

In contrast to these attitudes, EBM and clinical guidelines were viewed as useful tools to improve the quality of care. At the same time, physicians were suspicious that increased standardisation would threaten discretionary decision making. They called for "standards worked out by competent physicians' groups, standards that are not imposed from above but actually developed at the bottom" (FG 1, network, ambulatory care). The claims to define the standards of health care "from the bottom up" and "based on physicians' experience and practice", and the positive statements on quality management, were echoed in all interviews with members of quality circles. Strong resistance to regulatory tools applied "from above" was related to health policy, and, interestingly, also to physicians' own associations. Some participants added that bottom-up developed quality management provides a barrier against the influence of the pharmaceutical industry, which was characterised as coming "from outside".

The findings indicate that physicians promote elements of managerialism where professional power is strongest, while they reject those elements related to tighter public control of providers. In this situation, the emerging pattern of managerialism impacts on the organisational level but does not touch on the normative ground of medical power, namely self-regulation and the creation of a formalised knowledge system. The linkage of managerialism and professionalism – manifest in EBM, quality reports and clinical guidelines – provides physicians with new options to defend status and power and reassure trust. In contrast to an individualised marketisation, this linkage nurtures the search for a collective reference unit. Under conditions of rapid institutional and organisational change it is the biomedical knowledge system that provides a rather stable source of shared values, collective identity and practice, and professional power.

The search for collective strategies to defend physicians' interests continues when we look at networks; here, the most complex transformations of professionalisation enter the picture. Networking may be a response to increased competition within the profession enhanced by new health policies:

> "We are all engaged in a single combat, each of us isolated
> in our surgeries, so very isolated. And we feel the pressure,
> especially from outside, from politics, and this lack of trust
> in us and the loss of collegiality, and that is why we need
> the network." (FG 1, network, ambulatory care)

This dimension of individual support was also emphasised in all interviews with members of quality circles. Networks and quality circles thus cross the public–private divide of professional and individual interests. Besides the improvement of individual working conditions, improved quality of care through learning in peer groups and a critical review of their own practice in a confidential atmosphere were also major motives for networking. Physicians described cooperation and networking as a strategy to improve quality through 'creeping changes'.

They link different strategies of quality assurance via managerial tools, organisational change and sources of scientific and 'tacit' knowledge.

A third motive was maintenance of professional power. For example, quality circles were described as enabling "physicians to speak with one voice and act collectively" (quality circle, ambulatory care). In contrast to the improvement of the individual working situation and quality of care, the strengthening of collective power did not reflect a homogeneous attitude of quality circles but it was emphasised by the network of physicians in ambulatory care:

> "This shared trust also means that we can come together to present a common front to show those outside what's what, to show them the effort we put into our work, how good we are. Individually we can be beaten back, and when we can be beaten back we are easily convinced. This is one of the main reasons why solidarity amongst physicians is such a prized commodity." (FG 1, network, ambulatory care)

The 'common front' was defined as the cooperation of all physicians and all health care sectors; a balanced composition of generalists and specialists and equality of members were basic principles of this network. Cooperation of generalists and specialists, and office-based and hospital doctors was described as a "defence" against health policy attempts to divide physicians, and thereby weaken professional power. When it comes to the interests of SHI funds on single contracts with providers, the need to defend collective power was most pronounced – and sometimes described in the language of war. It was assumed that SHI funds would try to "break off" and "sell" individual physicians, and physicians therefore should present a "common front" to ward off such attempts:

> "The aim is not that physicians' networks should replace the associations, but we need a structure that shields us from them [SHI funds]. We don't have to reinvent the wheel but we must make it roll smoothly again." (FG 1, network, ambulatory care)

This statement underscores a finding from the survey, namely that the aim of network members is to transform – not replace – the corporatist structure (Chapter Five). Physicians feel the need to modernise self-regulation from the bottom up because associations, in their current form, were perceived as "encrusted" and governed by "stiff grandfathers" and "bureaucratic types", and therefore not capable of stimulating innovation, cooperation and collegiality. Networks thus seem to be the 'modernisers' of a corporatist system that suffers from old age and does not adequately respond to society's changing demands on health care, nor to physicians' calls on improved participation in a self-regulatory profession.

The emerging new strategy of professionalisation takes on classical elements of professional projects, such as collective professional identity, altruism and boundary work by the development of a common strategy – the 'front' against health policy and sickness funds. These familiar tactics are linked to new models of network governance and decentralised regulation. Although the hegemonic claims of physicians continue to exist, the 'front' is more hybrid and its boundaries, in some places, more permeable. Networks have the capacity to combine seemingly contradictory individual wishes for cooperation and self-determined work. They balance the power between individual and professional interests, scientific knowledge and embodied experience, between generalists and specialists, and between practitioners and the 'bureaucratic types' in the associations. In a situation where health policy reinforces competition but fails to target more inclusive patterns of professionalism, physicians develop their own models to coordinate the diverse interests of the medical profession.

Matching professionalism and managerialism: new strategies of trustful cooperation

Trust is a cornerstone of professionalism and a precondition of high-quality care (Kuhlmann, 2006b). A comparison of two provider networks studied here reveals that trust can be established in a number of different ways, and managerial tools provide new opportunities for trustworthy relations. The first example is a network comprising around 70 physicians – generalists and specialists – providing ambulatory care. In the second network a group of about 15 female professionals – mainly physicians from different specialties and also specialised psychologists – got together to improve breast cancer care. Both networks are regionally limited and chose the legal status of registered charities. Characteristic of both networks is that they began within regionally established structures based on shared aims of 'good care' for patients and the wish for cooperation.

In both networks the primary condition and basis for cooperation within a network was mutual trust, but the resources mobilised to build such trust clearly differ. The first network established new forms of active participation of all members in decision making, formalised rules and target setting on cooperation. Most importantly, it established a complex organisational structure to implement these rules and targets; this structure included plenary meetings of all members, various working groups on managerial as well as medical issues, and an executive board accountable to the members. The process of change was documented and monitored, for instance with scientific evaluations that took the provider and the user perspectives into account. Furthermore, a new model of documentation and patient information was developed and applied to all surgeries in the network. Advancement of clinical guidelines and EBM was also a common goal and theme of a specific working group.

While the cooperation of the female providers of breast cancer care was based on common quality standards, personal contact and mutual respect also played a major role. For example, next to high competence the main criteria for recruitment were trust in colleagues and existing personal relations. This caused a rigid exclusion strategy towards new colleagues interested in the network. Furthermore, this network did not introduce any sort of performance indicators or monitoring. And, after two years, the momentum for change in this group was running out of steam, in contrast to the network of physicians in ambulatory care that has created structural incentives for procedural regulation.

The findings reveal that managerial tools support effective networking and trustworthy relations, while trust built primarily on personal relationships and at emotional levels does not provide a sound, sustainable foundation. A positive impact of managerial tools on the physicians' working situation is especially visible when we look at contested areas of health care, such as physicians who provide care for drug users. A member of such a quality circle stated:

> "Personally, I greatly appreciate the clinical guidelines; they are of great help to us. When I started [with treating drug users] I took advice from two barristers in order to protect myself. That has become much better now. The debate on quality of care has helped to legitimise the work of physicians who provide services for drug users. It is important that this legitimation is continually strengthened, by the means of documentation, proof of evidence and efficiency." (quality circle, drug substitution)

This statement clearly confirms that classical elements of professionalism are matched with managerial approaches and scientific–bureaucratic medicine. This hybrid pattern of professionalism serves well to legitimise physicians' services and also fits the German system of 'strong judicial review' (Blank and Burau, 2004, p 35).

Challenge of integration to medical hegemony

The previous sections highlighted developments towards a more inclusive professionalism and, in this respect, confirm the picture of a profession more open to cooperation that emerged from the survey of physicians (Chapter Five). This section takes a closer look at cooperation between physicians and other health occupations; interprofessional dynamics are assessed with respect to the medical provider network and the multidisciplinary network of women's health care activists.

According to expert information from an SHI physicians' association, no multidisciplinary provider network exists in the region covered by my survey but several networks make provision for the possibility of cooperation with other health occupations. The network of physicians in ambulatory care studied here confirmed this information:

> "At first we thought that in two or three years we would end up with an organisation that included nurses, various social care services and physiotherapists. We have had offers, [...] but we are standing right at the beginning of the entire planning process[...]. At the moment we are just glad that we can cope with our work, we have enough to do." (FG 1, network, ambulatory care)

The aims of this network come close to a primary care model of integrated care (Chapter Two, this volume). However, physicians are not capable of putting this model into practice. Integration only proceeds with respect to surgery receptionists. Physicians have an interest in surgery receptionists identifying themselves with the network. Despite legal barriers the network members exchange surgery receptionists, especially the trainees, among individual practices in order to create a pool that can be flexibly employed. Surgery receptionists themselves have no say in exchanges of personnel between surgeries and are not involved in the planning; changes are driven by physicians' interests:

> "Now that labour costs are increasingly rising, we ask
> ourselves whether we could at least exchange the trainee
> surgery receptionist so that she gets a better education and
> exchange receptionists in situations like illness or maternity
> leave so that we have a pool of labour.[...] We haven't yet
> consulted the surgery receptionists. First of all we are
> working out the financial side of things.[...] With us, the
> trainee surgery receptionist is generally on the side of her
> employer. If she isn't, then she usually leaves the job." (FG 1,
> network, ambulatory care)

This statement clearly indicates that cooperation and networking
among physicians does not reduce hierarchy in the health workforce.
Moreover, receptionists are seen as potential buffers to rationalise
surgeries in order to improve the earnings of the surgery owner, and
physicians do not expect any significant resistance from the
receptionists.

Attitudes on multidisciplinary cooperation were more positive in
the network of women's health care activists. Participants in the group
discussion emphasised the need for integrated care with examples
from breast cancer care, and care for women who had experienced
violence. Although the organisational structure of the health system
does not support efforts towards integrated care, and rivalry exists
between professional groups, the women observed an increasing
openness of physicians in general care and hospitals, and also of the
SHI funds (Chapter Five, this volume). They expected further change
from inclusion of the users in the regulatory system:

> "When patients are more involved in the planning and
> shaping of health care then new impulses are brought in.
> New experiences would be brought in, new demands. And
> that would have a very favourable effect on integration."
> (FG 2, network, women's health)

Furthermore, the statements reveal the interplay between new health
policies and new opportunities for surgery receptionists. In the wake
of quality management and DMP, for example, surgery receptionists
are able to extend their competencies and take over new responsibilities:

> "And this greatly strengthens the self-esteem of surgery
> receptionists.[...] And a confident surgery receptionist could,
> for example, advise patients on nutrition in the DMP for

diabetes. Similarly, she could also extend her competence and the DMP could become interdisciplinary. There are chances here, no doubt about it." (FG 2, network, women's health)

A comparison of the two networks studied here reveals that improved cooperation driven by economic logic does not reduce hierarchy in health care. An extension of cooperation also calls for shared values and aims, like feminist approaches and the improvement of women's health care. Inclusion of health occupations and users, and teamwork approaches are essential elements of the women's health care movement (Kuhlmann and Kolip, 2005). Data do not reveal whether and how positive attitudes on integrated care actually translate into practice; and additional information from midwives confirm improved cooperation but tell a less favourable story of teamwork in the area of women's health care. However, the crucial point is that integrated care is a shared aim in the different groups of providers that is not based on short-term health policy incentives but nurtured by values, in this case, a strong commitment to women's health. The research underscores that changes in health care are driven by values rather than economic logic (Light, 1997; Chapter One, this volume). In this respect, it once again highlights the tensions between the currently dominant policy drivers (Chapter Three, this volume) and actor-based changes towards modernising health care that were explored from the data of the physicians' survey (Chapter Five, this volume).

Furthermore, the findings indicate that less hierarchical relations and cooperation with health occupations must be 'learned' and 'experienced'. However, the structure of the German health system – and the educational system, too – provides little opportunity to promote this process of learning. In this situation, positive impulses are arising from the efforts of physicians to advance interdisciplinary discussion and cooperation. The members of networks and quality circles gave several examples that shared values and interests may be extended to health occupations, and emphasised – "this calls for discussions to awaken understanding" (member of a quality circle, general care).

A changing pattern of professional identity is emerging that is based on trust and shared values and interests rather than simply on 'belonging to a club'. Similarly, the classic concept of 'autonomy' based on exclusion and hierarchy is remodelled in ways that allow for the inclusion of 'others'. For example, members of networks and quality circles emphasised a need for collegial discussions in order to "voice criticism" and "talk about difficulties without a loss of face"; these statements point to an increasing awareness of 'medical uncertainty' (Fox, 2002) that cannot be solved individually.

Medical identities are thereby becoming more fluid and contextualised. This tendency is especially visible when we look at the multidisciplinary network of women's health care activists. For example, a physician from this network emphasised the need for change in health care, which was expected to come from new managerial tools and improved participation of patients. Although she perceived the developments as challenges and sometimes even awkward for physicians, she acknowledged their contribution to positive changes to be more important than pressure on physicians. She made the criticism that physicians look at their own situation without assessing developments in context. For herself she was determined to: "revise my own limited perspective and take a good look at the wider situation" (FG 2, network, women's health). The emerging new patterns of cooperative and accountable professionals are an attempt to create medical identities under changing conditions. These new identities do not necessarily change the power relations but may further collaborative attitudes and the integration of new actors in the system of health care.

Quality circles and networks impact on institutional environments in positive ways and, in part, stimulate a move towards integrated care. However, no coherent 'learning system' is established to link these initiatives; health policy does not target the emerging potential for innovation. In this situation, as the most powerful actor the medical profession has the greatest opportunity to model and remodel health care according to its own interests.

Professionalisation of physiotherapy: travelling in a changing world of health care

Professionalisation of physiotherapy, in its former version, is a good example of inclusion by 'subordination' to the medical profession in terms of the typology described by Turner (1995). This occupational group is integrated in the SHI system, and many therapies physiotherapists provide are part of SHI care (Chapter Three, this volume). Patients need a prescription from a physician to get treatment, so this task is essentially delegated to physiotherapists by physicians. Physiotherapists have their own professional body but membership is not mandatory and they have not gained statutory self-regulation with full acknowledgement as independent stakeholders in the corporatist system. However, there are signs of change in this arrangement of subordination, and physiotherapy no longer fits neatly into the ideal types of professionalisation of health occupations.

Turner described three models of medical dominance over other health occupations, namely 'subordination, limitation and exclusion' (1995, p 138). These models relate to different strategies to gain professional status. 'Limitation' is a strategy to achieve professional status via containment for a specific therapeutic method or a specific part of the body; dentists, for example, applied this strategy successfully (Kuhlmann, 2001). 'Subordination' describes a situation in which the delegation of tasks by doctors is accepted. Inclusion in the health system is assured, but participation and self-determined work are limited. This strategy relates most closely to gender hierarchy and exclusionary tactics (Witz, 1992); the regulatory pattern is characterised as 'registering a difference' (Davies, 2002a, p 91). Saks points out that 'exclusion' as a third category is especially related to non-medically qualified alternative therapists, 'in which practitioners are denied formal registration altogether' (2003b, p 52). The following sections highlight that German physiotherapists are currently travelling between the borders of these ideal types and developing new tactics against a backdrop of changing institutional environments and demands on health care.

Professionalisation beyond subordination and exclusion

Physiotherapists accept formal subordination, while simultaneously searching for new options to free themselves from medical dominance and improve their market power and self-determination. They claim expertise for issues related to the physical functioning of the body and deny any competence of physicians in this area; this attitude of German physiotherapists is in line with international developments (Richardson, 1999). A physiotherapeutic approach is viewed as superior to biomedicine, especially in those areas where the limitations of orthodox medicine are most obvious:

> "I think that we are the experts in this area and that we should have the corresponding competence [to decide what therapy is used], and not prescribed by the physician who doesn't know [the details of] what he's writing on the prescription." (FG 4, university programme)

Members of the physiotherapy association echoed claims for independence and 'partnership' with doctors. The contradiction of formal subordination to physicians and an identity of being the 'real' expert, without, however, having the resources to translate this awareness into practice, provokes tensions and dynamics towards new strategies to better promote professional interests. A classic pattern of professionalisation via market control and state protection (Johnson, 1972; Larson, 1977) is not available under conditions of formal subordination, nor does this pattern accord with new demands on integration and participation in health care. In this situation, physiotherapists develop diverse and hybrid models. Classic elements, such as academic qualifications and market extension, are in part taken up and linked to individualised tactics of gaining market power.

Tactics of 'limitation' are most furthered by efforts to gain professional status via academic qualifications and inclusion in the university system. As described in Chapter Three, this strategy has made significant progress, but developments towards professionalisation are still limited. Physiotherapists lack a comprehensive formalised knowledge system and options to legitimise this knowledge. They currently lack the necessary academic qualification to develop scientific standards and give proof of evidence of their therapies; thus no system of quality management and public control is established. The crucial point is that the struggle for independence needs support from research that can only be carried out under the umbrella of physicians. Efforts to establish their own therapeutic approach, which is independent of and, in a limited area, superior to biomedicine, and to improve standardisation of knowledge and services are thus inevitably linked to subordination to the medical profession.

Further tensions exist within this occupational group. Material from the group discussions highlights that motives for academic training are devalued and interpreted as "they are no longer interested in working with patients" (FG 3, physiotherapy association). It was also stated that competition increases with the new career options, and this "naturally frightens a lot of people" (FG 3, physiotherapy association). The participants in new university programmes confirmed that they are often viewed with suspicion and treated as rivals. They feel marginalised and career routes for such pioneers for professionalisation are not yet determined:

> "I didn't think it would be so difficult to actually use the new skills and knowledge. And it's unbelievably frustrating that a Bachelor is really only a stepping stone. And now I'm working in a practice again as the physiotherapist. The Bachelor degree is a sort of mongrel, one starts the course

of studies with enthusiastic ideas, but nobody explains how
things will unfold later and what the possibilities are further
down the line or what my options will be." (FG 4, university
programme)

Although they complain about the lack of career pathways, the
participants in the university programme emphasised new options in
the wake of new organisational models, like DMPs, and new policies,
like the strengthening of prevention, patient-centred care, and quality
management. They had positive attitudes to clinical guidelines and
expected more 'objective' and 'transparent' criteria of decision making
that reduce the dominance of physicians: "I have more competence
and that means less dependence on the physician because clinical
guidelines exist that prescribe what has to be done" (FG 4, university
programme). Similarly, improved rights and participation of patients
were seen as promoting physiotherapists' independence from physicians:

"If there are more possibilities to explain things to
patients[...]. That patients then have a choice of what
treatment they want, and it's not just prescribed by the
physician." (FG 4, university programme)

The crucial point is that, for the time being, physiotherapists are
excluded from the development of these guidelines and programmes.
Physiotherapeutic care is not included in the evaluation of quality of
care; and no specific indicators or methods ensue from new policies
(Scharnetzky et al, 2004; Chapter Three, this volume). Furthermore,
physiotherapists do not compete with physicians on the level of patient
information and do not develop their own strategies to actively include
patients in decision making. The options for change are therefore
more of a vision to advance a professional project than a tool.

A further effort to improve occupational status relates to market
power and brings to the fore complex transformations in the system
of subordination enhanced from the bottom up by the practitioners.
Shifts are occurring in the relationship between doctors,
physiotherapists and patients. These transformations are furthered most
by the interest-based strategies of self-employed physiotherapists. They
are most obvious in the expanding areas related to fitness programmes
and health prevention, where a physiotherapist does not need delegation
from a physician and which are usually excluded from the SHI system.
Demand for such programmes continues to increase. Patients directly
contact a physiotherapist without seeing a doctor, and pay privately

for the service. Such strategies fit a category described as exclusion from the orthodox division of labour (Saks, 2003b). In this case, success or failure is regulated solely by the market. Tactics of 'exclusion' thus provide most opportunity for the powerful 'market-savvy' actors as fees are negotiated individually with the user, whose bargaining position is weaker than that of the SHI funds.

The growing importance of preventive care and its recent inclusion into Statutory Health allows for payment of some of these services by the sickness funds. In certain cases, the patient has to pay upfront and negotiate reimbursement with the SHI funds afterwards. This procedure deviates from the traditional structure of the SHI system, where fees are paid directly by the sickness funds to doctors or therapists and negotiated collectively with the representatives of the profession (Chapter Three). Although prevention is a minor part of physiotherapists' services and also marginal in SHI care, the new policies open doors to change the subordination and restriction to physicians' delegation. In the long run, the tactics of 'exclusion' could successfully translate into tactics of 'limitation'.

Attempts to transform and outflank subordination by expanding the provision of services that are excluded from SHI care are accompanied by a number of changes from 'within' the stakeholder arrangements and the expert–lay relationship. Physiotherapists are increasingly able to extend their scope for self-determined decisions; they make inroads as partners of patients, physicians and SHI funds. In focus group discussions physiotherapists reported that the diagnosis and prescription given by a doctor is sometimes changed; these decisions are made together with the patient without further consultations with the prescribing physician. In practice, the subordination to the medical profession is transformed 'laterally' in a way that advances the occupational control and self-determination of individual physiotherapists and the expansion of markets. Physiotherapists obviously have the power to undermine subordination, but fail to turn this power into a formal right, and physicians do not try to fully exercise control.

Physiotherapists confirm the findings on increased cooperation explored from the perspective of physicians (Chapter Five, this volume), and at the same time point to the limitations of this pattern of integration. Cooperation depends on the attitudes of individual doctors. Even if physiotherapists are fully informed and included in treatment decisions, this does not constitute shared decision making. For example, if physiotherapeutic treatment is recommended instead of surgery, "in the end the doctor decides and the patient is operated on" (FG 4, university programme).

Physiotherapists expected an upgrading of their occupational status from a stronger inclusion of patients in clinical decision making. However, patients are not perceived as collective stakeholders in the health system who might help to foster professionalisation, as they successfully did, for example, for midwives (Chapter One, this volume). Consequently, the alliance of physiotherapists and users may improve the individual working situation but it does not stimulate change in the regulatory system and the organisation of care.

Avoiding conflict: gendered tactics of professionalisation

With respect to professionalisation, individualised attempts to transform subordination are a highly precarious strategy. However, this strategy releases physiotherapists from both an increasing competition with physicians and collective responsibility for the provision of health care. The findings indicate that physiotherapists try to avoid conflict with the medical profession, and do not promote collective 'boundary work' against orthodox medicine and its representatives. It is interesting to note that none of the participants used the aggressive language observed in the group of physicians to call for social closure; physiotherapists want to establish a 'partnership' rather than a 'common front'.

With respect to market power, a subordinate position ensures protection of the medical profession, while a position as an independent stakeholder in the health system increases the risks of marketisation. Under conditions of cost containment and the increasing competition of providers, physiotherapists thus feel more comfortable in the niche of Statutory Health than as equal stakeholders with new commitments and accountability to patients, the public and their own occupational group:

> "We don't get the impression that there's a well-founded reason for the doctor's prescription. The reason why we still follow it is because we don't have the political clout to stand against the SHI funds. We don't have a situation where we can say we can do without the delegation [of patients] from physicians. This would quickly result in the sickness funds saying, 'then we'll take you out of Statutory Health and reimbursement altogether'. And the public hasn't yet arrived at the point where the patient would come directly to us and say, 'I'll pay the fee out of my own pocket', or call

for reimbursement from their sickness funds." (FG 3, physiotherapy association)

The findings confirm that physiotherapists lack state support and market power, on the one hand, and occupational closure to successfully apply a classic strategy of 'limitation', on the other. In this situation, the tactics of 'limitation' may easily turn into 'exclusion', and thus into a status of non-medically qualified practitioners. Such a status would enhance deprofessionalisation and does not, therefore, appeal to the majority of physiotherapists. The physiotherapists' association also considered their own list of tariffs for physiotherapy, similar to that established for midwives. But this was also rejected as a 'risky option' under conditions of cost containment and lack of professional power.

Physiotherapists' claims to independence and participation are highly ambiguous and nurtured by different and even contradictory interests. In this situation, new strategies are emerging that move beyond 'exclusion' and 'limitation'. The efforts to improve status are based on individual negotiations on work rather than classic elements of professionalisation through formal rights and statutory self-regulation. Subsequently, the results are less certain and less stable. In the long run these tactics may turn out to be precarious with respect to the professionalisation of physiotherapy as they do not provide a solid foundation for sustainable collective action and identity.

The efforts towards professionalisation are characterised by an overall lack of legalistic tactics. This result points towards intersections between professionalisation and gender in an occupational field with about 80% women. The strategies show striking similarities to the historical struggle of German women to gain access to the professions, which is typified by a lack of legalistic tactics (Kuhlmann, 2001). It is interesting to recall here Witz's (1992) historical analysis of female professional projects that explore legalistic tactics as more successful than 'credentialism' (Chapter One, this volume). The strategies adopted by physiotherapists – regardless of whether male or female actors – seem to be governed by nation-specific gendered tactics to achieve professional status.

Group discussions with members of the association reveal an even more complex interplay between gender and professionalisation. Physiotherapy was characterised as a 'women-friendly' occupation, which provides the most opportunity to combine work and caring responsibilities. This is especially true for physiotherapists in ambulatory care, where part-time work is a common working pattern. Members of the association reported that female physiotherapists achieved upward social mobility through marriage rather than improvement of their own occupational status. Part-time work in physiotherapy is not sufficient to 'bring home the bacon', and the German welfare system supports a 'male breadwinner model' (Lewis, 2002). Subsequently, the women accept low earnings and limited career options. They invest more energy in the actual therapeutic work with patients than in improving professional status and collective power. Both the members of the association and the academic physiotherapists complained strongly about the general lack of interest in professional politics. Physiotherapists were seen by them to be "sitting in a warm nest and afraid that something could change" (FG 3, physiotherapy association).

The common attitude was characterised as "me and my patient", as one participant (FG 3, physiotherapy association) put it. This means that physiotherapists limit their scope of action to the individual therapeutic situation. The potential for advancing the professional project of physiotherapy is thus limited, and interest-based strategies are gender biased. Individualised tactics of extension of services into markets not protected by Statutory Health are most furthered by the group of self-employed physiotherapists with higher quotas of men (Chapter Three, this volume), while the participants in the university programmes – mostly women – apply more classic strategies of professionalisation through academic acknowledgement. They deviate, however, from a gendered pattern of professional work and identity – related to working with patients – and thus travel along a road without signposts.

Different roads towards professionalisation

Physiotherapists themselves create an identity of 'professional workers', offering high-quality health services that differ from those provided by other professions. Even if professionalisation does not lead to an improvement of occupational status, the belief in the power of professionalism is in itself an engine for change. Professionalism emerges as an altruistic 'mission' to establish a physiotherapeutic approach independent of medicine and to further change in health care. The participants in university programmes felt an urgent need for action regardless of individual benefit. This altruistic logic fits well with the common attitudes of physiotherapists. Economic logic was characterised as somewhat "unmannerly" for physiotherapists (FG 3, physiotherapy association). The academic physiotherapists put more store by their work as professionals than on financial aspects, thus transforming an identity of 'me and my patient' to 'my profession and me'.

The innovative aspect is that these participants refer to professionalism and collective identity without necessarily taking over the tactics of exclusion embedded in classic professionalisation. Boundary work is still alive but in a process of redefinition. It is interesting to note that integration, multidisciplinary working styles, and patient-centred caring models are being used as a discourse to advance professionalisation and define physiotherapy as different from the medical and nursing profession. Like the physicians who work in networks, academic physiotherapists wish for collective power, occupational independence and cooperation. However, they are constructing more permeable boundaries and developing new concepts of professionalism that recognise the value of the qualification of other health care workers, teamwork and communication (Hüter-Becker, 1999; ZIPT, 2005). For example, the university professors of physiotherapy are currently improving cooperation with other therapeutic occupations, particularly occupational therapists, and discussing an interdisciplinary university programme.

Furthermore, physiotherapists create an identity as 'change agents' who are in line with the demands of a changing health policy and best serve the needs of patients. According to this identity, accountability, public control and improved rights of and information for patients are welcomed as tools that advance the professional project. Similarly, physiotherapists see quality management and the improvement of preventive care as occupational chances. These fields are perceived as more open for new actors because demand for them is fairly recent and the medical profession has had less time to occupy the arena. Here, physiotherapists apply tactics that aim for transformations of professionalism 'from within' (Evetts, 2003), even though they lack the power and resources of the medical profession.

Overall, we can say that physiotherapists are exploring various new paths towards professionalisation. They accept and even welcome the exclusion from the SHI system in a particular area of service, where their state licence and professionalised status enhance market power and trust of the users in their services. Nonetheless, with respect to the services that are included in Statutory Health and where they are subordinated to physicians, they are still struggling for participation and self-determination. Their demands for self-determined work are particularly supported by changes in the health care system; they may also be furthered by the medical profession itself, which increasingly cooperates with physiotherapists as partners in a limited area of health services.

Processes under way go beyond classic strategies of professionalisation and point to flexible arrangements between the tactics of 'exclusion', 'subordination', and 'limitation'. The most complex dynamics are enhanced through academic qualification, which closely relates to tactics of 'limitation'. This is the most contested area as the efforts run counter to the interests of powerful actors in the field of physiotherapy; firstly, those of self-employed physiotherapists who promote strategies of individualised marketisation, and, secondly, the schools of physiotherapy that defend a traditional educational system and a market monopoly against university programmes. Academic qualification also goes against the grain of the dominant gendered pattern of action and identity, and hereby increases competition and rivalry within physiotherapy.

In this situation, the need increases for coordination and negotiation of diverse interests. The associations do not adequately fulfil these demands. Participants in university programmes and expert information make clear that there is increasing dissatisfaction and even frustration with the physiotherapy associations. In this respect, physiotherapy mirrors developments in the medical profession (Chapter Five, this volume) and an overall loss of trust in the institutions in society at large. However, there are important differences to physicians' attitudes and strategies. In particular, the academically trained physiotherapists complained about the absence of collective strategies that actively take on new demands in health care:

> "The association has not taken a clear position, that clinical guidelines and evidence-based medicine are necessary in order to maintain an independent occupational group in future [...] and that the association does not really support academic training [...]. The problem lies much deeper [...] that there is absolutely no agreed understanding of this occupation, so there is nothing like an occupational identity in physiotherapy." (FG 4, university programme)

A further issue was that regional physiotherapy associations competed instead of collaborating, so physiotherapy speaks with many voices. Findings from the focus group with members of a regional physiotherapists' association confirm this assumption. However, attempts towards collective action are under way at a federal level with the establishment in 2005, for instance, of a new working group on professionalisation. More radical change and innovation can also be expected from a new federal-level initiative of academic physiotherapists and practitioners called 'Future Initiative' (ZIPT, 2005; Chapter Three, this volume). This initiative applies tools from network governance and open coordination. Membership is open to all physiotherapists who share the aim of professionalisation, including members of the physiotherapy associations. Attempts to improve cooperation and coordination reflect similar developments in the medical profession. However, the network initiative of physiotherapists is not linked to organisational change and provider models, and nor does it aim at statutory self-regulation.

In conclusion, we see that physiotherapists apply diverse strategies to change their status of subordination to physicians. The varieties of strategies can be viewed as an attempt to advance the transition from an occupation to a profession under conditions where classical tactics are not available, and professional interests are becoming more heterogeneous. Interest-based tactics of exclusion are still alive within the occupational field, and at the same time, new patterns of a more inclusive professionalism are emerging. However, the contribution to both the modernisation of health care and the promotion of a professional project is restricted: a gendered pattern of professionalisation is not adequately linked to formal rights and statutory self-regulation; and the state does not support the efforts towards an independent profession and a more inclusive pattern of professionalism.

Surgery receptionist: women's struggle for self-determined work in a subordinate position

The surgery receptionists in the study confirmed the picture that was drawn from the physicians' network: they are 'objects' of physicians' governance rather than 'subjects' in a changing system of health care. In addition, the findings bring to the fore a negative impact of the regulatory framework on the occupational situation of surgery receptionists that new health policies may even reinforce. The receptionists complained bitterly of their exclusion from the regulatory system and lack of acknowledgement:

> "We're just not taken into account in the health care reforms, and we are not perceived as belonging to an independent occupational group. If someone talks about a hospital, everyone knows there are doctors, nurses, the

different occupational groups are relatively clear, but this is not the case in ambulatory care." (FG 6, receptionists' association)

Subordination and lack of agency continue at the micro-level of work. In the discussions receptionists complained that their working times were not adhered to; they often had no regulated lunch breaks and overtime was the norm rather than the exception, in some cases without overtime pay or days off in compensation. Owing to the long working hours of physicians (Chapter Five, this volume), receptionists are expected to work as long as doctors deem to be necessary:

"We work under constant pressure. And I know that if I don't get this done now I'll be working until 9 pm and won't get home until 10 pm.[...] I'll still have to be here again at 8 am in the morning. You can't leave before you've finished your work. My boss is quite open about it and says, 'My surgery receptionists have to be flexible and be prepared to work overtime because that is what this surgery needs. And if you can't cope with it...'." (FG 5, training programme)

While in many occupations flexible working hours improve the work–life balance, and thereby the career options, especially for women with caring responsibilities, in health care increased flexibility actually leads to the opposite, and even worsens the situation for surgery receptionists. Doctors apply the logic of lean management and see receptionists as a means of rationalisation. They react to an expected or actual financial loss with wage cuts or firing surgery receptionists instead of improving efficiency and quality of work, for instance by introducing teamwork approaches.

Participants in the focus groups confirmed that doctors' attitudes to quality management were in general positive, but not related to quality of staff and the training of surgery receptionists. Critique reveals an overall deficit in physicians' competencies to 'manage' a surgery, and organise work and staff. Changes in the surgery are not linked to new tasks and opportunities for the receptionists. In this situation, workload and occupational dissatisfaction increase – leading to a negatively charged working atmosphere and more frequent illness. As one participant put it: "We are constantly under stress and work our fingers to the bone. We are ill more often; there is nothing you can do about it" (FG 6, receptionists' association). It is interesting to note that those who worked in surgeries where team meetings took place and a communicative organisational culture prevailed were more satisfied with their working and training conditions than those without such teamwork approaches.

Although team meetings were highly valued, none of the participants reported attempts to call for team meetings or to introduce meetings of the receptionists to improve communication. Furthermore, rationalisation increases the pressure on the receptionists to accept unfavourable working conditions and even significant cuts in already low wages for fear of unemployment. Such concerns are warranted given Germany's high unemployment rate and the low market value of surgery receptionists' qualifications. Subsequently, dependency on the practice owner and rivalry between surgery receptionists increases, making them even more vulnerable to coercive demands from their employer.

Lacking all the key resources, such as state protection, market control, academic training and a formalised knowledge system, surgery receptionists cannot apply classic tactics of professionalisation. They have only very limited options at hand to improve self-determination and upgrade occupational status. Under these conditions, their struggle focuses more on better individual working conditions than on control of an occupational field and market.

Governing surgery receptionists: the merger of professionalism and gender

Doctors make use of two powerful order patterns to govern their staff. They refer to professionalism and an altruistic ethos to serve patients' needs whenever necessary, and they rely on gendered attitudes that silence the receptionists and reduce resistance. "Of course we're fulfilling a typical woman's role and accept whatever's thrown at us, that's often the case", is the way members of the receptionists' association described the problem (FG 6, receptionists' association). This gendered attitude is not specific to Germany but reinforced, firstly, by a health political culture of 'familialism' and 'subsidiarity' (Dent, 2003; Blank and Burau, 2004). Secondly, married receptionists are less dependent on their earnings (due to the German income tax system that favours a 'male breadwinner model') and thus often do not resist low wages and may even accept wage cuts. The vicious circle observed in physiotherapy is even stronger in the case of surgery receptionists: low occupational status and lack of career chances together with a lack of more enabling welfare state incentives for labour market participation of (married) women cause an ongoing 'blockade' of collective action.

Furthermore, surgery receptionists develop an occupational identity that is inevitably linked to 'their' doctor; this was already visible in the group of young receptionists after three years of training. A participant in the focus group characterised the attitude as "my doctor and me" (FG 6, receptionists' association), and interestingly, the work situation was sometimes even described as "we're like a family". In the case of surgery receptionists, the limitations of an occupational identity are not based on 'work with patients' as in physiotherapy, but on 'work with doctors'. The effects are even worse: the 'reference unit' of surgery receptionists is the medical profession, often reduced to an individual practice owner. The strategy of surgery receptionists can best be characterised in terms of feminist theories that highlight the social construction of gender and the active role of women in these processes: surgery receptionists are 'doing gender' (West and Zimmerman, 1991) while doing work and thus 'doing deference' according to the needs of doctors and patients. The merger of professionalism and a traditional gender order seems to be a perfect tool in the hands of physicians to assure subordination and govern surgery receptionists, even in times of gender equality.

The discourse of professionalism is imposed on surgery receptionists, and at the same time the receptionists in the study referred to professionalism to claim acknowledgement of their work and independence from doctors. They took on an altruistic ethic of physicians and considered the maxim: "Enjoy the work and don't look upon it as just a job" (FG 6, receptionists' association) to be an important prerequisite for a qualified receptionist; and they related the struggle for acknowledgement "to commit fully from one's own sense of duty" (FG 6). Nevertheless, they complained of the gap between formal rights and actual competencies; one participant described the situation as "being treated like a little schoolgirl" (FG 6). In contrast to their powerless position, the receptionists claimed professional competencies that are important for the future health workforce:

> "Surgery receptionists today aren't just there to say, 'next patient please'. We work on sophisticated medical equipment and we're there to offer professional services [to patients], and, and, and…. And they [doctors and health policy makers] still haven't got it, that this is what will be

important in surgeries in future." (FG 6, receptionists' association)

Participants were well aware that they are needed by doctors. If a receptionist strictly confined her work to her formal tasks, "the doctor couldn't 'process' 100 patients a day.[...] The doctor is nothing without the surgery receptionist, we prepare everything" (FG 6, receptionists' association). The crucial point is that this identity of a 'professional worker' does not translate into incentives for doctors and nor does it impact on health policy. Rather than fighting for their rights, surgery receptionists set their hopes on a 'turn for the better' and on support from 'others', like doctors and patients: "The most important part for us would really be if the patient would stand up and say 'not with me'" (FG 6, receptionists' association). It is interesting that this call for action and resistance is not related to the receptionists themselves. A passive attitude of 'complaining but not acting', which was also present in physiotherapy, is much stronger here. In contrast to physiotherapists, the receptionists do not even apply 'credentialist tactics' (Witz, 1992) but just 'delegate' strategies to further occupational interests, and avoid any conflict with doctors.

Once again, gender identity is a serious barrier towards surgery receptionists taking on a more active role in health care. One important reason for their tolerance and passive attitude is a feeling of being responsible for 'their' doctor. For example, a participant reported she was looking for a new job following a wage cut: "But then I say to myself and my colleagues, 'just go and leave him in the lurch, now...?'" (FG 6, receptionists' association). This statement highlights that demanding better working conditions was perceived as contradicting moral responsibilities of 'caring' for others. According to this attitude, gender identity – caring for others – clashes with strategies of gaining benefit from self-determined action independent of physicians and contradictory to their interests. Professionalisation strategies refer to occupational 'interests' but surgery receptionists refer to 'private' responsibilities. Consequently, professionalisations strategies do not touch on this level of conflict or provide options to improve agency.

Searching for self-determination without advancing a professional project

Members of the receptionists' association developed clear demands on self-determined work and a future vision of the position of receptionists in the surgery:

"The job description of a surgery receptionist, or whatever we might be called in future, has to be totally separated from the medical profession. We have to arrive at a point where we can make autonomous use of the skills and knowledge we acquire during training [...] no more delegated tasks. A surgery receptionist must be able to practise what she's trained to do [...] have possibilities of independent work within the surgery. It could be nutritional adviser, for instance, something one could really do oneself, independently." (FG 6, receptionists' association)

Surgery receptionists lack the power to translate their demands for self-determined working conditions into occupational change. They fail to develop any collective strategy to improve occupational status and market control, although there is a tendency to imitate physicians' tactics of professionalisation. For example, specialisation is already on offer for surgery receptionists in radiology. And the participants in the study, especially those in the training programme, called for further options according to medical specialty. In contrast to the medical profession, this strategy does not relate to market control. Moreover, specialisation and intraprofessional differentiation impact negatively on labour market chances as the scope of competencies and options are understandably narrowed down. In this situation, the only way out for many receptionists seems to be a change of occupation. Half of the participants in the training programme stated that, given a second chance, they would not choose this occupation again, and about a third were either planning to look for other options or were already actively searching.

In addition to a high turnover rate we can identify other tactics that fit the category of 'exclusion'. On the whole, surgery receptionists welcomed health policy attempts to extend tailored services and out-of-pocket payment as this provides new opportunities for self-employment; a growing demand for courses in nutrition, in particular, was seen as a new chance. They also mentioned their competencies in management and documentation as an option for self-employment. The stumbling block here is that this strategy calls for a high level of self-initiative and competencies to compete in an unprotected market with other health occupations that have better qualifications, such as nurses, dieticians and psychotherapists, who enjoy higher levels of public trust. This may be one reason why more experienced receptionists, but none of the participants in the training programme, mentioned self-employment as a new option.

In terms of the categories developed by Turner (1995), individualised 'exclusion' tactics may, in the long run, undermine 'subordination'. Members of the receptionists' association characterised the health reforms as a "job machine for future surgery receptionists" (FG 6). New occupational fields are emerging, especially in the area of quality management, documentation and health prevention. To a great extent, chances for surgery receptionists in these areas depend on the strategies of other players: the response of doctors to managerialism, demands of the service users, and health policy decisions on inclusion of new services in SHI care.

Changes in health care nurture the vision of self-determined work and status improvement but the mechanics of the 'job machine' may easily relegate surgery receptionists once again to the bottom of the health workforce. For example, hospitals increasingly employ surgery receptionists in order to reduce costs. Here, receptionists replace the more expensive nurses, but this does not necessarily lead to upward mobility. As in ambulatory care, hospitals use the women as a means of rationalising staff without offering new career options. Policy changes do not translate into a professional project, and do not even improve individual working conditions. Surgery receptionists attempt to gain more self-determined working conditions without 'boundary work' with physicians and other health occupations. In contrast to physiotherapy, no professional association or network is on the horizon that could successfully promote the interests of surgery receptionists.

The crucial point is that neither health policy nor user groups support the attempts of surgery receptionists to make use of the 'job machine'. While physiotherapists are manoeuvring with high flexibility 'within' and 'outside' SHI care and responding to user demands, surgery receptionists surrender to new markets that are not yet fully developed, highly contested and more dependent on demand of the medical profession.

Deceptive appeal of professionalism and the need for state regulation

In the case of surgery receptionists the appeal of professionalism is a deceptive one. A deception, moreover, that makes them subject to doctors' governance while nurturing the illusion of being part of a professional system that might, possibly, include the receptionist. The findings indicate that some doctors are aware of the competencies of receptionists and confirm an increase in teamwork approaches as described by physicians themselves (Chapter Five, this volume).

However, as we have seen, the power of physicians to define cooperation is much stronger than in physiotherapy owing, for example, to the strategy of exchanging receptionists between physicians working in a provider network.

Where attempts to utilise professionalism as a facilitator of occupational change clash with actual working conditions and career perspectives – because the surgery owner does not belong to the group of innovating doctors who value the work of surgery receptionists – changing jobs to a different occupation often seems to be the only way out for the receptionist. Job dissatisfaction is reinforced as disappointment with the occupational situation spills over into personal relations – inherent in the image of the surgery as 'the family'. In this situation, the options of collective action to upgrade occupational status and the chances offered by changing health policies disappear into thin air.

An important potential for innovation has been woefully neglected with respect to modernising ambulatory care. The findings make clear that even the participants in the training programme were able to identify the weak points in the management and organisation of work in their surgery. Their suggestions to improve surgery management included teamwork, regular meetings, improved communication between the receptionists and between doctors and staff and better working hours regulation. Deficits in communication and collaboration were key issues of critique and job dissatisfaction. Given that dissatisfaction of staff and lack of collaboration and coordination of work have a negative impact on the quality of care, there is an urgent need for action. Furthermore, increasing rationalisation of surgeries through reduction of staff negatively impacts on patient communication:

> "When I'm my own [at work], I don't have time to talk to the patients. Many of them come to the surgery just to meet us and to talk about something. Lots of them live alone.[...] But I just don't have any more time." (FG 6, receptionists' association)

The analysis of deficits and proposals for change are well in line with the demands on modernising ambulatory care (Chapter Three, this volume) but surgery receptionists themselves do not have the power to bring about innovation. A traditional gender identity and gendered division of labour that puts women's work at the bottom are serious barriers to the active promotion of occupational interests. Although physicians' awareness of the competencies of surgery receptionists might be on the increase, it is not to be expected that they will voluntarily relinquish powerful tools with which they can govern staff. In this situation, state protection and inclusion of surgery receptionists in the regulatory system of corporatist stakeholders would simultaneously promote the occupational situation of the receptionists and the efficiency of the health care system.

Towards varieties of professionalism: challenges for coordination

This chapter has highlighted transformations of professionalism on different levels and in different occupational groups. The findings indicate an increasing diversity and new patterns of professionalism that enhance dynamics towards a more flexible and inclusive professionalism, however slight these shifts may be at present. Professionalism thus serves well as 'facilitator' of modernising health care that is capable of including new logics, like managerialism, and new demands on professions, like cooperation and integration. A changing order of professionalism is applied to the entire field of health care but utilised in different ways. One characteristic feature is an increasing need for new strategies of interest-based occupational politics and a redefinition of 'social closure'. Tensions between strategies of exclusion embedded in professionalisation and new demands on inclusion are reinforced, for instance, when service users enter the picture, or integrated caring concepts call for a collaborative health workforce.

The three occupational groups studied here hold different positions in the health workforce and regulatory system and differ significantly as far as power, social status and resources are concerned. They are all, however, manoeuvring to position themselves in a changing arena of health care and searching for new options to assure or upgrade status. Classic patterns of professionalisation – such as statutory self-regulation, market control and state protection – continue to be important, but a seemingly stable ground of professional power is increasingly becoming dynamic. In this situation, individualised tactics of improving market power are gaining ground. These tactics tend to increase the power gaps within and between professions and occupations, and run counter to both the aims of professionalisation and those of modernising health care. At the same time, new models of network governance are emerging that balance diversity of interests and further cooperation.

Changing health care systems thus enhance diverse and contradictory sets of dynamics (Chapter Five).

Whether and how the emerging spheres of opportunity can be used to assure or gain professional power depends on the stakeholder position of the actors in the regulatory system and a gendered pattern of professionalisation. The state and its model to govern professions is an essential issue for the success or failure of professional projects, but changes in health care cannot be explained without taking gender into account. Developments in physiotherapy and also in the field of surgery receptionists reflect a gender order that spills over into the occupational field. This order is embodied by the occupational players, and embedded in health policy and institutional regulation. Accordingly, gendering the actors of professional projects (Witz, 1992) does not go far enough, and must be extended to include a gender-sensitive approach in the regulatory framework. The two occupational groups studied here highlight that the impact of gender stretches far beyond disadvantages of women and so-called female occupations in the health labour market. Moreover, results point towards serious barriers for the modernisation of health care. There is no sign that new health policies will actually reduce these barriers or result in a collaborative health workforce.

In this situation, dynamics are enhanced, initially and most importantly, within the various health occupations and the medical profession. The observed transformations of professionalism do not replace medical hegemony and paternalism but move beyond the lines of division in the health system, namely gender, generalists and specialists, providers and users, as well as professions and allied occupations. These developments may provoke shifts in the balance of power in health care, which are most obvious in the medical profession. However, there are also weak signs of interprofessional dynamics. Dynamics from physicians' networking and more inclusive patterns of professionalism may spill over to the health occupations and also to the service users. The crucial point is whether the emerging network culture of physicians and the advancement of cooperation and coordination translate into a 'learning system' that is capable of transforming its own professional boundaries.

Health policy neither supports nor targets the development of such a learning system of integration. The exclusion of health occupations from the joint self-regulation of Statutory Health and the absence of any particular regulatory body for the health occupations are serious barriers to modernisation in Germany. The result is a systematic lack of coordination in interprofessional dynamics, or even changes in a single occupational field. Furthermore, change in professional strategies and identities is not adequately linked to institutional change and not stimulated by macro-level regulation. Neither the health care nor the educational system in Germany is prepared for the new demands on coordination, integrated care and teamwork.

There is a need for comprehensive regulation of the entire health workforce that is not governed by physicians' interests and SHI funds, but subject to public interests and control. It is such a model of regulation that would contribute to citizenship and modernisation of health care, and target the translation of new patterns of professionalism into varieties of 'citizen professionals'.

SEVEN

New actors enter the stage: the silent voices of consumers in the landscape of biomedicine

When 'citizen consumers' fall ill, we can test the promises of new governance and citizenship. We can study the tensions between the new demands arising from the inclusion of users – as citizens, consumers and patients – in decision making and the interest-based strategies of the professions, especially medicine. This chapter brings in the patients' perspectives. Do patients take on the role of expert patient? Does the model actually serve their demands and needs? Does it provoke shifts in the system of care? And how does the medical profession react to claims for user participation? Changes are analysed on meso and micro-levels: the informed consent and shared decision making of patients and doctors, and the new procedures of formalisation and standardisation of care via EBM and clinical guidelines. Results show that the medical profession is capable of transformations that include new demands. A consumerist model of a market-savvy expert patient thus challenges medical power and knowledge without necessarily shifting the balance of power. Data highlight that patients are willing to exercise their new role as experts in some situations, while wishing for help and advice in others. Tensions are thus embedded in the model of a citizen consumer, who is expected to take over self-responsibility for health and exercise control over providers. These new tensions may turn out to challenge the government rather than the medical profession.

Power and partnership: the deceptive promises of consumerism

The move towards consumerism is connected to new promises of partnership between users and providers, especially doctors, and the inclusion of user representatives in the health policy process. Health policy calls for 'self-responsible' citizens, and attempts to shift the balance of power towards service users in order to improve the control of providers. However, the promises of participation do not translate easily into changing power relations and more 'empowering' conditions of health care. The limitations and obstacles can be identified on different levels: a lack of institutional support and organisational strength of user initiatives; the diversity and ambivalence of patient demands and wishes; and the reflexivity of medical practice that is capable of including and transforming new demands on partnership with patients.

Health policy increasingly includes user representatives as stakeholders on regulatory boards. Recent changes in the public law institutions and the legal framework of health care described in Chapter Three mark an important step towards improved citizenship rights in the area of health care. However, at present, the users are "second-class stakeholders" – as one representative put it – who lack the resources to exercise their new role of controlling providers. Often, SHI funds and physicians' associations do not take them seriously and they are not fully informed. The negotiations on the DMPs, for instance, reveal further disadvantages that are caused by the regulatory system itself: all information on these programmes has to be treated confidentially and external expertise is not allowed during the negotiation process. Accordingly, a user representative has to collect all information alone – or break the rules – while physicians and SHI funds can rely on a wealth of expertise from their own institutions.

The crucial point is that user groups are not prepared for their new governing responsibilities. No bottom-up democratic structure exists that would allow for legitimised user statements on health policy. Widely different service users are forced to speak with a single voice, and decisions strongly depend on the personal attitude and competencies of a specific representative. The top-down strategy of participation is not accompanied by health policy efforts to improve the organisational coherence of various user representatives and patients' self-help groups. The government does not provide the resources to improve coordination and negotiation of user interests.

In this situation, attempts to influence user groups are increasing, especially on the part of the pharmaceutical industry. The focus group discussions, in particular with the diabetes and breast cancer groups, reveal a number of such attempts. For instance, pharmaceutical companies often invite members of self-help groups for conferences, meetings and information classes – and pay for all expenses – where information is given on new drugs and therapeutic options. In general, the participants in my study welcomed this additional source of information and were uncritical of the interest of the pharmaceutical industry to use self-help groups in order to open up or protect markets.

Some participants even expressed an attitude of being taken seriously as self-responsible 'consumers' and 'expert patients'.

With respect to the political level of decision making, one user group representative reported that some representatives enjoy their new role as "VIP" and the status attached to "belonging to a powerful group" of decision makers, and tended to forget that they were speaking for patients. He criticised the government for not providing the necessary financial resources and legal requirements to develop an organisational structure of independent user groups that would reduce the power gap in the regulatory system, and serve as a barrier to various forms of corruption.

The patients in the self-help groups I consulted for my study echoed complaints about lack of resources. The participants actively take up the discourse of consumerism. They are willing to exercise self-responsibility and make informed decisions but made new demands on the government to provide better information and improved access:

> "I can't encourage people to take self-responsibility seriously and tell them that they should be more aware of health issues if, at the same time, I close avenues of information or don't even open them up.[...] And at the moment I see a great discrepancy here. You can't call for self-responsibility and tell people that they should be informed while simultaneously giving them no realistic chance to obtain information." (FG 7, self-help group, coronary heart disease (CHD))

It is interesting to note that patients do not restrict the new demands on self-responsibility and exercising control to the medical profession but extend this new role to the government itself. They wish for state control and legal rules on health care information. Participants suggested, for example, the establishment of "an official national institution open to all concerned, an independent technical supervising organisation" similar to that responsible for the technical control of vehicles (FG 9, self-help group, breast cancer).

Data reveal that patients do not believe that the SHI funds function as such a controlling institution and are highly suspicious of any attempts of these funds to improve user information. All group discussions highlight patients' lack of confidence and significant dissatisfaction with the SHI funds, which tend to be more interested in saving costs than in quality of care and patients' wishes. Although SHI funds significantly improve patient information, for instance through call centres, all focus groups complained of a lack of information and transparency. Participants were also highly critical of the quality of this information and the competencies of SHI funds. By contrast, trust in 'their own' physician was much higher; I will come back to this issue in the next chapter. Participants expressed more sympathy for doctors working under extreme time pressure – especially in the hospitals – and budget constraints in ambulatory care than for SHI funds.

Patients perceive a contradiction between a policy discourse of participation and actual health policy, which does not adequately target the improvement of transparency and the provision of reliable information. The DMPs CAMe in for heavy criticism. The patients in the study felt they were mere 'objects' of these programmes and had no part in decision making. The comments on the DMPs reveal an overall anxiety that opportunities for self-determined decisions will be reduced rather than increased: "It makes you wonder what they [government] are going to do with us" (FG 11, self-help group, diabetes), or, "Once you're in a system like that, everything just takes its course" (FG 10, self-help group, breast cancer). Further queries stemmed from the continuous increase in patients' out-of-pocket payments, even for treatments that patients perceive as medically necessary and useful. All groups complained about such increases, which are perceived as unfair and as 'punishing' the patient for being ill.

Uncertainty and negative attitudes about the new programmes are not surprising, as none of the patient groups – although themselves the target of these programmes – had easy access to clear information. For example, one participant in the breast cancer group had collected information from the Internet in order to prepare for the group discussion. Regarding the diabetes programme – the first to be implemented – a few patients had received leaflets from their SHI funds but said they did not contain what they wanted to know. None of the members of the CHD groups had received any information. One participant reported that she had asked her SHI fund for information but was still waiting for an answer after nearly a year, and another expressed the opinion that, "the SHI funds do not welcome patients who ask questions" (FG 9, self-help group, breast cancer).

Political demands call on physicians to improve transparency and patient information, but the health policies introduced to effect this are not transparent for patients. Rather than better chances of participation, patients perceive a loss of options for self-determined decision making. Key demands are the freedom to choose a physician and individually negotiate on the diagnostic procedure and treatment, and the reimbursement of all treatments by the SHI funds. Patients perceive this 'freedom of choice', which is traditionally guaranteed by the SHI system, as the most important condition of self-determination and self-responsibility. It is precisely here, however, that freedom will be restricted, to avoid 'doctor hopping' and to reduce health care expenditure. The perceived contradictions between promises and practice nurture patients' negative attitudes and dissatisfaction with new health policies and the government. Patients may also form new alliances with doctors against the government and SHI funds. This is likely to happen where the interests of patients coincide with those of physicians – or specific groups of physicians – to avoid tighter regulation and standardisation of care, and organisational shifts towards a gatekeeper system.

The government has largely failed to address the concerns of 'the spirits it has summoned' – the citizen consumers and expert patients, bold and savvy enough to claim their rights. The findings from the group discussions reveal that patients expect the government to improve the control and coordination of services and access to information:

> "It would be wonderful if there was a help centre that I could go to right from the start.[...] I don't think it's right that I have to scratch around by myself for the information I need. And if I'm not careful then I draw the short straw."
> (FG 10, self-help group, breast cancer)

Patients are willing to take responsibility for their own health, at least in part, but expect the government to take responsibility for the functioning of the health care system and to provide an enabling context. The findings highlight tensions between the government's expectations of the user as a stakeholder in the regulatory system and the demands of patients on state responsibility for health care. These tensions may hasten the decline of trust in the state and its institutions. Even new regulatory models with a positive impact on patient participation, like the DMPs, are viewed with suspicion. Patients felt themselves to be 'objects' rather than actors in the health care system.

The 'expert patient': a new generation of patients

Data from the Health Monitor Survey reveal that patients wish for a more active role, but not one that is necessarily linked to control of providers. About half the participants in this survey "did not simply want to be well informed, but also wanted to bring their own individual perspectives into diagnostic and therapeutic decisions" (Isfort et al, 2004, p 89). Above all, patients perceived the advantage of additional information from the Internet as a way to better understand issues of health and illness and change their own behaviour; control of doctors played only a secondary role (Isfort et al, 2004, p 96).

These results indicate that the advancement of expert patients does not necessarily lead to increasing conflict with doctors. Moreover, these developments point to shifts in the attitudes of patients to more self-responsibility that mirror society's move towards individualisation and changing modes of citizenship, particularly social inclusion and participation (Chapter One, this volume). It is interesting to note that a change in patients' attitudes is not necessarily perceived as threatening by health care providers either, but as a move towards partnership:

> "Patients have changed. There's a new generation that doesn't want to be bureaucratically administered from the top down, but says, 'We can only move forward with power and partnership'. Not confrontation but partnership. This is largely music for the future, it hasn't happened yet. But I can already hear the instruments tuning up." (FG 2, network, women's health)

The findings from the focus groups with patients provide deeper insights into the advancement of this new generation of patients and its demands and strategies. Analysis shows that patients not only want information but also criteria that enable them to judge the quality of that information. They do not expect an individual doctor to know everything, but feel a certain degree of self-responsibility and try to collect pertinent information from a variety of sources. Patients wish to seek the counsel of other people outside the patient–physician relationship, for instance via telephone counselling. This wish for multiple sources of information is not, however, an expression of mistrust in physicians. Moreover, those who felt best informed generally placed high levels of trust in their doctors. Although the participants in the focus groups reported a number of examples of wrong treatment decisions or lack of information, they do not wish this to be interpreted as mistrust in their own physician. They simply want the option of additional, independent sources of information:

> "So that one can also ask a question without running the risk of insulting one's own doctor. That one doesn't have to name them. I mean so that one can ask a question without

having to give the name of one's own doctor. Just to express one's own doubts. I would find it a super idea. And perhaps it would even strengthen some people's trust in their own doctor." (FG 7, self-help group, CHD)

In order to improve communication with doctors they take their role as expert patients seriously and prepare for their appointment by reading books, asking advice of friends and self-help groups, or searching the Internet. "You have to educate yourself" (FG 11, self-help group, diabetes), was a common attitude. Further strategies are: "I make a note beforehand of all the questions I want to ask" (FG 8, self-help group, CHD). Being accompanied by a partner was also reported to be a helpful strategy, but one that, it was often said, the doctor viewed with suspicion.

A strong desire to be well prepared for a doctor's visit was observed in all groups. Controversy remained, however, about the 'duty' of patients to gather information themselves beforehand. Discussions with participants in the CHD and breast cancer groups – and also diabetes type I – generally placed more emphasis on self-responsibility for collecting comprehensive information. Compared to these groups, a consumerist attitude was weaker in the diabetes type II groups, where the average age of participants was significantly higher than in the others. The findings mirror differences related to age, also reported in other studies (Isfort et al, 2004).

A further issue that touches self-responsibility was health prevention. CHD groups, in particular, showed a high level of motivation for preventive action, and called for better information in order to improve individual behaviour. Patients with diabetes type I expressed similar attitudes. Here we can assume that a public discourse on risk factors for CHD and diabetes related to lifestyle impacts on the attitudes and behaviour of patients. The women in the breast cancer group were also highly motivated for lifestyle changes and prevention but complained of a lack of scientific knowledge on the reasons and risk factors for breast cancer. Here, self-responsibility and prevention were more related to physical exercise, physiotherapeutic advice and alternative therapies; I will come back to this issue later. Compared to the CHD and breast cancer groups, attitudes on prevention and self-responsibility for lifestyle changes were less positive in the self-help groups for diabetes type II. These differences may also be an outcome of age-related attitudes.

Taken together the findings do indeed point to the advancement of a new generation of patients that takes responsibility for its own health.

These patients see better information and knowledge about their illness and the various treatment options – especially preventive health care – to be important prerequisites of self-responsibility. On the whole, they are willing to exercise their new role as 'citizen consumers' with both rights and duties but they are not equally willing to do the job of controlling providers.

Claiming self-determination and seeking help: the ambivalence of an expert patient role

Patients' demands for self-determination and information are growing but remain highly ambivalent. In their new role as active consumers, patients often feel subjectively unable to cope. In some situations, they wish for a doctor's help and advice. The tensions between self-responsibility and dependency on doctors' advice and information were an important theme in all group discussions. Both men and women highlighted this dilemma but the women in the breast cancer groups most clearly outlined the conflict:

> "That one really has to take on an active role. And if you're not able to, then you don't get the best care, I mean the wide spectrum that you're entitled to.[…] You only get what you explicitly ask for. You don't get it automatically. You have to struggle with everyone – with the insurer, the doctors. You have to find out, who is the specialist and how do I find him.[…] It has to be improved so that one can choose what information one is flooded with. And one does not have to cope with it all alone because, often, one just isn't able to." (FG 9, self-help group, breast cancer)

Notably, even patients who are well educated and well informed felt that it was expecting too much of them to always behave according to the model of an expert patient and consumer. In a particular situation they seek doctors' advice for what it is necessary to know. Several participants in the group discussions described situations where they felt "totally alone", "at the mercy of the system" and helpless:

> "That you're in such a weak position as the patient, and you need all your strength just to get through this treatment [chemotherapy]. And that you just aren't capable of claiming your rights and making sure that you get what's best for

you. You really need support from the outside for everything." (FG 10, self-help group, breast cancer)

The logic of consumerism calls for an independent actor, capable of claiming his or her rights and clearly stating his or her demands. However, this logic clashes with the 'real world' and the wishes of severely ill patients:

> "In this situation, I can't ask any questions at all.[...] If I had gone myself and said, 'I'd like to discuss it', then it would probably have been all right. But in this situation I was just glad to get out again. That's the end of it [chemotherapy], I don't want a discussion now!" (FG 9, self-help group, breast cancer)

The ambivalence of the role of an expert patient, and the tensions between the wishes for self-determination and support from others are not unique to German patients or the health care system. For example, similar results are reported in an Australian study (Lupton, 1997) and an evaluation of the NHS Direct service for health care users in the UK (O'Cathain et al, 2005). It is interesting to note here that the patients in my study redefined 'freedom of choice' to mean help and advice from physicians and others. 'Choice' is not merely perceived as an individual action, but set in context and even connected to notions of paternalism: doctors are expected to select information, as patients are not able to cope with a flood of information. 'Self-determination' and 'autonomy' are thereby becoming more contextualised concepts that are open to the inclusion of 'others'.

It is no mere coincidence that the ambivalence of an expert patient role was most apparent in the breast cancer groups that emphasised the wish for help in a particular situation, without, however, accepting the classic paternalist behaviour of physicians. Gender identity allows women but not men to articulate a wish for help. Men also reported situations where they felt helpless, but this was usually restricted to a single situation and immediately followed by an example of agency and power. The advent of expert patients reinforces a gendered coping strategy of men that does not allow for feeling helpless and seeking support from others. The tensions between seeking help and claiming expertise may therefore play out differently for men and women.

The wish for alternative therapies and the reluctant power of biomedicine

Participants in the patient groups claimed access to comprehensive information, including information on alternative therapies and services carried out by other than medical providers. In general, they made the criticism that information is limited to biomedical issues, although "other things play a part and that there might be alternatives; there's nothing in school medicine about that" (FG 13, self-help group, diabetes type I). It is worth noting here that the physiotherapists in the study reported that physicians do not adequately inform patients on alternative options, thus limiting patients' choices to biomedical treatment (Chapter Six, this volume).

All groups in the study called for more information over the entire spectrum of health care. However, the CHD groups emphasised classic areas of prevention, like physical exercise or non-smoking programmes and diet, rather than alternative treatments. In contrast to this, demands for alternative and complementary services were generally more pronounced in the breast cancer groups and the diabetes type I group. The differences between the groups reflect different conditions and treatment options related to the illness but they are also an outcome of gender differences. Members of the women's health care network reported that, "women are more interested in getting information on complementary treatments and psychotherapy" (FG 2, network, women's health). Participants in the breast cancer groups confirmed this assumption: "That's what I really miss, any sort of psychosocial care. There was nothing at all" (FG 10, self-help group, breast cancer). A further important issue was the lack of physiotherapeutic services and information on health prevention, especially physical exercise.

Several women reported that they had consulted alternative practitioners, especially homeopaths and naturopaths, after biomedical treatment had failed to help them. They outlined the particular benefits of alternative therapies for chronic conditions and called for their inclusion in Statutory Health. For example, one woman in the diabetes type I group said she had had problems with her stomach for years. She had undergone numerous diagnostic procedures to identify the underlying bacterial cause, but no therapeutic intervention had alleviated her pain:

> "I then had to go to an alternative practitioner with non-medical qualifications (*Heilpraktiker*). I had to pay it all myself, but afterwards it got better. I don't agree with it

[biomedicine], I had to swallow so much poison and nothing helped until I went to the alternative practitioner, but the sickness funds didn't pay for this." (FG 13, self-help group, diabetes type I)

The lack of information on CAM and exclusion of these therapies from SHI care was one of patients' major complaints, but this criticism does not tell the whole story of biomedical power. A statement from the breast cancer group highlights the subtle interplay of medical knowledge and individual beliefs in this knowledge:

"And I have to admit that they [doctors] are all very helpful and tell me things. Even when I didn't understand, they took their time and were patient and explained it to me. There is just one thing that shook me. If you don't want it [chemotherapy and radiation], if you don't want to be pumped full of poison [...] then you're really left alone because there's nowhere else to get information. I asked the insurers if they could give me an idea of how much they would pay towards alternative therapies. They didn't understand what I wanted.[...] And what got to me even more is that you're no longer a human being. You're a tumour that has to be treated. And then you get chemotherapy and radiation and drugs. And if you don't want that then you don't fit into the system and the standards, and then it's better if you leave and don't show yourself there anymore." (FG 10, self-help group, breast cancer)

Despite her strong and well-informed negative attitude to chemical and radiation therapy, this patient had felt unable to resist the pressure, and thus decided to accept radiation therapy: "Because I thought that I might not be able to come through it alone and then I would worry about whether I'd made the right decision". Paradoxically, in summing up, she emphasised the positive experiences with physicians' information: "Up until now my experience hasn't been of the worst Someone was always there when I needed somebody".

This example highlights the gap between information given by physicians and the demands, needs and wishes of patients. At the same time, it points to the 'seeping' of medical knowledge into individual perceptions and fears. Patients are quite capable, at least to a certain extent, of developing their own ideas of quality of care that deviate from those of the medical profession. However, they are not capable in each particular situation to fully reject the definitions of biomedicine.

The growing interest in CAM sits side by side with trust in doctors and biomedicine. However, patients' awareness and actual experience of the limitations of biomedicine – especially to treat chronic illness – challenge both the medical profession and health policy. It is interesting to note that patients tend to complain more about the non-reimbursement of alternative treatment by the SHI funds than about physicians' information. They were also critical of a health policy that does not include the entire spectrum of health care services in Statutory Health and does not provide comprehensive information. Tensions between patients' increasing interest in CAM and the promises of health policy to improve consumer power provoke yet more dynamics in the system of care. While physicians increasingly react to user demands by offering preventive care and alternative therapies – paid for by patients themselves and thereby strengthening the market power of the medical profession – SHI funds and health policy are not well prepared to meet the changing demands of the service user.

Information: the new line of division in health care

The patient groups studied here highlight that patients generally feel that they get the necessary information from their doctors provided they are well informed and able to put their questions in the right language at the right time and to the right physician. Patients with a high level of education, access to alternative sources of information and financial resources have new chances to participate in decision making. The situation was compared to "a bazaar, where everything must be negotiated, and success depends on the individual power of the patient" (FG 10, self-help group, breast cancer). A new social divide stemming from differences in access to information was especially emphasised in the CHD and breast cancer groups; Internet access was crucial in obtaining information on health care and different treatment options:

> "Not everyone who falls ill has an academic education, and not everyone can use the Internet.[...] What happens to the women who have neither the power nor the capability of taking their own treatment in hand?" (FG 9, self-help group, breast cancer)

Similarly, a participant in the CHD group said he feels "inferior and not very articulate" and thus not able to negotiate with physicians. This statement highlights the fact that improved information is only one condition in the empowerment of patients; the capacity to communicate competently and the tenacity to see a situation through are equally relevant. These competencies are heavily biased towards patients who are well educated and have high socioeconomic status.

Social differences between patients are reinforced by physicians' practices. A previous study of hospital doctors revealed that a patient's social status impacts on physicians' decisions and information. Although doctors claim to treat patients equally, medical practice is in fact shaped by social influences. Against a backdrop of scarce resources, such factors are becoming increasingly important. Doctors in this study confirmed that, generally, the more demanding a patient was, the better the information he or she received:

> The patients at the greatest disadvantage are those in poor social circumstances and who can't express themselves either. Patients, who can't defend themselves, namely those with chronic conditions or the elderly, are left behind. (cited in Kuhlmann, 1998, pp 47-8)

In line with these findings, participants in the self-help groups assumed that patients from low-income groups are not informed about therapeutic options excluded from SHI care, while patients who are able to pay for alternative therapies themselves get more comprehensive information.

While consumerism fosters inclusion processes, it does so at the expense of all social groups that are not 'market-savvy' and cannot communicate effectively. The statements – both from the provider and the user side – bring into view that anyone who is weak in the processes of negotiation – socially or because of age or temporary serious illness – is at a disadvantage. A new pattern of exclusionary tactics via information produces social inequality, which is legitimised by the 'autonomous' decision making of physicians and 'freedom of choice' of market-savvy patients. A 'citizen consumer' model causes a shift in responsibility from the macro-political level of welfare state policies to the micro-political level of users and providers of health care services. Existing social differences and the inequality of patients are thus treated as an individual problem rather than a societal concern.

These developments indicate an important shift in German health policy away from the historically developed principle of compulsory health care and social solidarity towards marketisation. The findings reveal that patients are highly critical of these shifting relations, and call for health care responsibilities to be carried by society as a whole. While health policy creates a homogeneous image of self-determined users acting in a 'rational' and self-responsible manner, it fails to deal adequately with both the diversity of patients' needs and wants and the existing social inequalities.

Shifting the balance of power in the expert–lay relationship

Calls for 'informed consent' and 'shared decision making' of patients and physicians have unleashed a decisive process of change in medical ethics (Kuhlmann, 1999). The findings of the survey confirm that physicians translate new demands for patient participation into practice. As described at length in Chapter Five, the vast majority is willing to improve patient information and work in partnership with patients. In contrast to this changing pattern of professional practice, however, a negative attitude on patient rights was observed in the profession as a whole. Of the physicians surveyed, 83% did not consider that improved patient rights serve the new demands on health care: 50% expected no effect and 33% even a negative or very negative impact (5-point Likert scale). Asked for a dichotomous ranking (important/ less important) of conditions of high quality of care, the figure is only slightly more positive: only 31% of the surveyed physicians judged 'improved patient rights' as important.

Physicians further participatory practices in an area where their power is strongest, namely the micro-level of physician–patient interaction, but oppose patient participation when it comes to statutory rights. The new logics of informed consent and partnership thus complement but do not replace paternalist attitudes. A previous study (Kuhlmann, 1999) carried out with doctors working in hospitals provides deeper insights into physicians' attitudes and practice of patient information:

> As the consultant physician one is always tempted to minimise something or not be completely frank, or even lie. This is partly an attempt – whether wrongly or rightly, it doesn't matter – to save the patient anxiety or to avoid a problem oneself. This temptation, to get rid of a time-consuming problem, was always with us. But it has become increasingly easy to succumb to it due to increasing time pressures. (cited in Kuhlmann, 1999, p 69)

Informed consent remains a fairly limited option to improve patient participation as long as information lies in the hands of the medical profession. Doctors often desist from fully informing patients, if the economic interest of the organisation and medical ethics are contradictory. They fail to disclose the financial constraints underlying medical decisions in order to avoid conflict. Doctors are well aware of their monopoly on information and their power to influence patients' decisions:

> I can inform the patient comprehensively, but one still wants to target him or her towards a certain treatment. One can point out alternatives, but one mustn't forget that one would like to lead the patient in a certain direction. (cited in Kuhlmann, 1999, p 74)

The patients in my present study highlighted further limitations of partnership and shared decision making. In the case of serious illness and acute need of care, patients are not able to review medical information critically:

> "There is a lot of work to be done with explaining and educating. But then, when you're ill yourself you can't start questioning things; you just aren't capable. If you don't have someone who supports you, someone to whom you can say, 'Please come and help me' – and who has that anyway – you can't find things out by yourself. And it doesn't matter which hospital you go to. If you don't question things yourself, the doctors just think they'll do what they have to do. They prescribe chemotherapy and assume that you know all about it." (FG 9, self-help group, breast cancer)

The participants in the focus groups confirm that some doctors take patients' wishes and lay knowledge seriously, but many others do not. Patients perceived the time pressure of physicians as a serious barrier to adequate information and shared decision making. At the same time, they showed great understanding for the time constraints of physicians. In all groups participants cited examples where physicians had taken time to talk to patients, despite heavy workloads, and some who even offered information classes in their free time. Similarly, there was disagreement in all group discussions as to whether or not doctors treat patients as partners. A negative example was usually followed by a positive comment on doctors' attitudes on shared decision making and self-determination of patients. Criticism was levelled more at a system of health care that lacked coordination, and deficiencies in the surgery management, than at individual doctors.

At the same time, all group discussions highlight that doctors are inherently unable to handle criticism. Subsequently, patients often do not tell their doctor about information from other sources. One participant stated, "you have to pretend to be stupid, so that the doctor isn't offended" (FG 8, self-help group, CHD). Another reported that he "was treated like a greenhorn" (FG 8, self-help group, CHD). By contrast, patients have a strong desire to "talk openly" (FG 13, self-help group, diabetes) and would like their own experience and observations to be taken seriously.

It is interesting to note that patients perceived a change in professional attitudes and behaviour in the younger generation of doctors. Several participants reported that younger doctors take the individual experience of patients and lay knowledge more seriously than their older colleagues. This observation corresponds to the findings of the survey of physicians, where younger age predicts slightly more positive attitudes to patient rights (Chapter Five, this volume). In addition, the previously mentioned study on decision making of hospital doctors also points to more positive attitudes of the younger generation regarding the self-determination of patients and full disclosure of medical decisions (Kuhlmann, 1998).

However, demographic change in the medical profession does not necessarily shift the balance of power in health care. The interviews and group discussions with physicians reveal that changing attitudes of patients are accompanied by new strategies of physicians; especially, networking and cooperation can be used to defend expert power against patient participation in decision making: "That was a motivation for me to ask myself whether we couldn't cooperate a little bit, otherwise the patient does what he wants with us" (FG 1, network, ambulatory care). Similarly, a member of a quality circle stated that these circles improve the "self-esteem [of doctors] and a self-assured manner with the patients" (quality circle, general care). Another physician confirmed that "quality circles can also improve competence in dealing with difficult questions and patients" (quality circle, drug substitution). It is interesting to recall here that membership of a network does not further more positive attitudes on patient rights (Chapter Five, this volume).

A very different attitude was manifest in the group discussion with the network of women's health care activists. Here, patients were perceived as 'change agents' of the health system and partners in health care:

> "Patients are becoming more self-aware. And when things are no longer paid by SHI care, then they go to the sickness funds and make trouble.[...] I think it's coming now [change], like in the '70s when the women started to stand up, something could really change from the bottom up in health care. It's a new movement, I really do think so." (FG 2, network, women's health)

The results point to increasing heterogeneity in physicians' attitudes to the role of patients in health care decision making. Whether and how patients are treated as partners depends on the individual physician. Under these conditions, the freedom to choose a physician and exit a therapeutic relationship is becoming even more important. This, in turn, may strengthen patients' demands for 'free choice' and clash with health policy attempts to introduce a gatekeeper system. Furthermore, the findings give proof of the transformability of professionalism (Chapter Six, this volume). Patients are included as new actors in the system of care without, however, substantively changing the rules and rights to define health care according to biomedicine and the interests of physicians.

Information as a 'one-way road' from physicians to patients

Even where physicians consider patient information to be an important component of quality of care, improvement focuses on formal procedures. The physicians in a network for ambulatory care studied here improved access to information through leaflets and a comprehensive collection of personal patient data that was handed over to the patient. Physicians thus clearly contribute to the expansion of information but there is very little evidence for diversity of information. Similar to the results reported from other health care systems, German physicians treat information primarily as a 'transfer' action, and only seldom as a process of 'exchange' (Lee and Garvin, 2003, p 449; see Sullivan, 2003; Bissell et al, 2004).

This pattern of biomedical-centred information does not fit well with the needs and wishes of patients. For example, participants in the diabetes type I group said that numerous training courses on nutrition and insulin therapy are offered and paid for by the SHI funds, but that these courses do not adequately take the circumstances and attitudes of patients into account. Behavioural advice and counselling on insulin treatment are modelled on artificial and ideal-typical life conditions, and thus failed in everyday life. Physicians are partially aware of these problems but often feel unable to offer individual counselling, due to time constraints. For example, in times of personnel shortages and budget constraints, hospitals offer group education for patients with diabetes in order to fulfil the formal requirements (Kuhlmann, 1999). In contrast to this, the patients in the focus groups wished for more contextualised information that fits their individual demands.

Furthermore, patients seldom complained about lack of information from physicians, but were more concerned about questions that do not fit the biomedical standards: "Then [the doctor] lets down the shutter and the conversation comes to an abrupt end" (FG 7, self-help group, CHD). Other participants reinforced this statement with comments like: "Yes, because they're not sure of the matter, otherwise they could have answered" (FG 7, self-help group, CHD). Patients take the role of generalists as gatekeepers seriously, and call for a more holistic style of information covering the entire range of care. They expect more comprehensive information, especially from the providers of general care. However, the findings of the physicians' survey do not indicate that generalists are willing to respond to this; the physicians in general care had slightly less favourable attitudes to patient rights and improved patient information in their own surgery than specialists (Chapter Five, this volume).

In contrast to patients' demands, for the main part information is reduced to orthodox medical knowledge and therapies. The question of what patients want to know is not addressed, only what they *ought* to know in order to play their roles as 'informed partners'. This dilemma is especially visible in the DMPs that, while attempting to improve information and quality of care, do not include patients' perspectives as a source of information and knowledge (Chapter Three, this volume). One participant described the situation as follows:

> "They [doctors] do explain a little. You sit there for a half an hour; then you leave, get an information sheet to take with you. And then you can read it. But that is all." (FG 9, self-help group, breast cancer)

The findings indicate that few doctors take the self-knowledge of patients and diagnosis resulting from self-examinations seriously. Several participants reported that doctors dismiss patients' own diabetes and blood coagulation checks. The women in the breast cancer groups highlighted further problems of doctors' attitudes. They complained of stereotyped images on women with breast cancer, which leads to a dismissal of the worries of those women who do not fit the stereotypes. Primarily, this problem concerns young women with children, as the typical patient at risk for breast cancer is an older woman.

Information and communication continues to be a 'one-way-road' from physicians to patients. Patients are 'educated' according to the interests of physicians rather than 'enabled' to make informed decisions that fit their individual lifestyles and attitudes on health. Under these conditions, the increasing call for evidence-based information may even reinforce the tensions between the demands of patients and the provision of care that is defined according to biomedical evidence.

Ambivalence of standardisation

Standardisation of care is a key strategy to improve quality of care and to enable patients to assess provider services (Chapters Two and Three). Overall, the patients in the study welcomed performance indicators, quality reports and evidence-based information as helpful tools to make self-determined decisions possible. At the same time, they are suspicious of standards and guidelines. They fear a reduction to a single standardised model, regardless of individual demands and needs. This fear was expressed in all groups and made up an important part of the discussions. It also brings to the fore a critical and often very negative attitude to health policy and institutions, especially SHI funds:

> "What happens if we sign a contract [to participate in the DMP]? What happens to our data? And will we still have our standard regime and then only get three control strips [for diabetes] a day? This worries me, I really do worry about that [...] then there is only a given standard, I think this would be bad.[...] Insurers only care about getting money for their contracts [from public funding for DMPs]."
> (FG 11, self-help group, diabetes)

From the perspective of patients, information, transparency and 'rational' criteria for quality assessment open up pathways to deal with uncertainty and to gain a measure of control in clinical decision making. The possibility to make decisions based on transparent criteria is perceived as a prerequisite for building trust and taking a more active role in decision making. However, information alone does not really cover the demands of patients, and an overall scepticism to new health policies is not merely a result of lack of information on new models of care. Instead, the ambivalence of patients' perceptions of scientific-bureaucratic measurements of medicine mirrors the problems and deficits of EBM and currently dominant models of standardisation.

Patients were highly critical of the biomedical bias manifest in moves towards standards and clinical guidelines. They emphasised that standards do not cover the entire spectrum of health care needs; in particular, "standards do not say much about quality of communication" (FG 10, self-help group, breast cancer). It is interesting to note that the worries about the limitations of standards were often mentioned with regard to complementary therapies – like regular courses of physical exercise in the CHD groups, or physiotherapy and psychotherapeutic counselling in the breast cancer groups – rather than in connection with the core areas of biomedical care. Furthermore, increasing standardisation and the advocacy of EBM as the 'gold standard' of care clashes with the demands of patients for self-determined decisions:

> "But in the end it's up to me to decide and say, 'all right, perhaps it isn't scientifically sound, it's still not a standard, perhaps it's still being studied. But I choose this way quite consciously because it's my way [...] because I have faith in it, because I think it helps me'. And so I should also have the possibility of using it myself." (FG 9, self-help group, breast cancer)

The ambivalence of standardisation and a one-size-fits-all model is especially visible in the breast cancer group. The women welcomed clinical guidelines and defined standards of care as tools to reduce unwarranted variations, to control physicians and to reduce negotiations with SHI funds on reimbursement. They expected an improvement of quality of care through standardisation, and at the same time, expressed worries and fears that standardisation reduces freedom of choice and neglects individual needs and wishes. The statement of a young woman in the breast cancer group demonstrates most clearly the ambivalence to standardisation. She reported that she was treated according to "an elderly-women-standard in breast cancer care". Her self-knowledge and her demands were not taken seriously; and in the situation of acute illness she was not able to fight with SHI funds for an adequate diagnosis and treatment. She now faces serious disability and a loss of quality of life:

"It really worries me [standardisation] because I think we have had [the experience] of the illness right from the beginning. And then they come, people who don't have the special knowledge that we've acquired. And then they want to tell me what treatment I must have; and they twist my arm again and tell me what I must and mustn't do. I think it's bad. Of course, this contradicts a bit what I said before about if there are standards […] but you have to look very carefully and see who sets up these standards."
(FG 9, self-help group, breast cancer)

The ambivalence of patients' attitudes to standardisation impacts more generally on the attitudes on DMPs and nurtures scepticism to new health policies:

"Of course, one hopes that they [DMPs] will improve quality. But my fear is that this is not their aim; that all possible kinds of interests lie behind them. Perhaps reducing costs. And everyone brings in their own particular interest, only we patients are hardly a part of it.[...] I'm very afraid, and I'm very sceptical." (FG 9, self-help group, breast cancer)

If standardisation is viewed through the 'lens' of patients, the deficits become apparent. In its current version, standards are heavily biased towards biomedicine and expert knowledge, while the perspectives of patients remain marginal. The efforts to define standards of care fail to cater to the diversity of needs and demands. Asymmetry in health care continues as long as patients – and other than biomedical providers of health care – are excluded or remain marginal in the negotiations of standards.

Moving beyond the market-savvy reflexive actor

Listening to the voices of patients brings home the ambivalence and limitations of a 'citizen consumer' model. The findings indicate that patients actively take up the discourse of consumerism and claim expertise and self-determination in health care, but in various ways and with demands and strategies that may even run counter to health policy. Patients redefine and transform a consumerist model. Similar to the developments in the medical profession, improved user participation is not merely a new policy but a complex and uneven process of social change. Once again, we find actor-based changes and different sets of dynamics that do not necessarily point in the same direction (Chapter Five, this volume).

Improved information and the new instruments of assessment offer patients a way to judge the quality of care beyond their individual experiences, and to make more self-determined decisions. The entrenched paternalism of the medical profession is not thereby automatically abrogated. It does, however, come under pressure to legitimise itself if patients have additional information at their disposal with which to judge the quality of a provider and biomedical services. This legitimation cannot be provided merely by more information or improved access and better evidence of patient information. Moreover, patients call for *other* than orthodox medical information and *other* than technological communication of information that is sensitive to their individual needs, demands and wishes. This means that new methodological challenges have to be met to amalgamate individual perceptions and scientific measures, and orthodox and alternative knowledge systems. Up until now, however, physicians have managed, by and large, to stonewall these demands (Chapter Six, this volume), and health policy does not increase the capability of patients to exercise their new role as experts more effectively.

A 'new generation of expert patients' does not radically replace medical power but releases new dynamics in the system of care and the health political process. Although user representatives are marginal in the joint self-administration of SHI care, an interplay between improved user rights and the growing interest of patients in CAM, together with their demands for the cooperation of providers and a more holistic model of care, may impact from the bottom up; these developments may provoke change in the organisation and content of health care. Improved user participation may thus release dynamics even in those areas that were identified as switchboards of change and knots of power (Chapter Four, this volume). However, it is not very likely that a consumerist model of user participation will actually shift the balance of power in the corporatist stakeholder arrangement.

My findings indicate that the government cannot rely on patients as partners to control health care providers. Even where new models of care improve transparency of services and control of providers, these efforts are viewed with suspicion and overshadowed by the worries of patients. New promises of participation and the better control and transparency of care clash with the actual experiences of patients. Health policy creates and nurtures new hopes for patients but does not adequately serve their demands. Tensions are thus reinforced between state responsibility for health care and the self-responsibility of patients.

A consumer model of participation neglects patients' wishes for help and support in some situations; it also creates new social inequalities in health care. This results in the continual disappointment of patients and an increasing loss of confidence in the institutions and the state, but not necessarily a loss of trust in physicians.

Patients do not act as micro-level governing agents or 'discriminating consumers', and consequently, they challenge the market logic embedded in new health policies. Patients create their own model of a context-dependent 'citizen patient', who makes self-determined decisions *and* seeks out doctors' help and advice, and who claims equality of care and state responsibility for the health of its citizens. This model moves beyond the logic of a market-savvy reflexive actor. Tensions between health policy and the interests of patients are especially visible when it comes to the role of SHI funds in the regulatory arrangement. The findings clearly indicate that patients do not perceive sickness funds as partners that speak for patients. From their perspective, SHI funds are organisations that follow the economic logic of maximising profit and therefore act as a constraint on both patients and physicians. Against the backdrop of these perceptions, it should not be expected that patients support the attempts of health policy to shift the power in favour of SHI funds.

A core idea of the Bismarckian SHI system – namely to delegate user interests to SHI funds and ensure democratic rights and participation of users through election of representatives of SHI funds – is perhaps more undermined by the mistrust of patients in these institutions than by an increasing marketisation and change in the regulatory system. Similar to physicians who value self-regulation but claim a more active role in the regulatory processes of the profession, patients call for more active participation in health care decision making. Patients amalgamate the normative promises and cultural values of a Bismarckian model of social security and equality in health care with a 'modernised agenda' of freedom of choice, participation and self-determination. This amalgamation creates ongoing dynamics and – as the alliances between the users, the professions and the state are not predictable – may enhance new instabilities in the health care system.

If the government expects the service users to do the job of governing and controlling providers, it should be aware that users might extend this job to health policy itself and challenge state regulation. In this situation, professions are increasingly needed as mediators between the state and the citizens in order to win back trust in the government and public law institutions and to gain stability of regulation.

Part III
The rise of a new professionalism in late modernity

The third part of this book investigates cultural order patterns as the connection links between professions, the state and the public (research design step IV; see Figure i.1). Two key categories of professionalism serve to explore the mediating role of professions and reflexivity of change: namely, trust and knowledge. Both categories are cornerstones of professional power and also of the functioning of societies, which undergo significant change. The empirical findings presented in the previous chapters are linked to an international debate on the governance of health care and changing modes of citizenship. Results highlight that 'information', 'freedom of choice' and 'autonomy' – the promises of modernity – are embedded in new models of governance and medical practice. The developments enhance complex shifts in the balance of power in health care that move beyond the impact of marketisation and bureaucratic regulation and the discourse on consumerism. The tensions between elements from new governance and conservative forces of medical dominance give rise to new and more diverse patterns of professionalism in late modernity. These new patterns open windows of opportunity for the improved participation of citizens and accountability of professions without, however, radically reducing the power of the medical profession to shape and reshape these processes of change.

EIGHT

Professions and trust: new technologies of building trust in medical services

Professions play a key role in building trust in the provision of health care. At the same time, the capacity of professional self-regulation to serve the interests of the public and to ensure the quality and safety of health care has come under scrutiny. This chapter highlights new perspectives in the debate on trust in health care. Instead of simply echoing the ideological complaints of the medical profession on the potentially adverse effects of the tighter control of providers, it brings into view new 'technologies' of building trust. This approach directs attention towards the intersections and tensions between changing patterns of governing the health professions and the new 'signifiers' of trustworthiness, which are based on tools from NPM. Both physicians and service users are increasingly demanding transparency and 'rational' criteria to prove the trustworthiness of providers. I argue that the information metaphor serves to amalgamate the call for the control of providers and the desire to seek trust in medical services. It is a key component in new technologies of trust building and the 'bridge' between the various actors and diverse interests in health care. The crucial point is that this bridge is constructed following the blueprint of the biomedical knowledge system. At the same time, it opens up pathways for changes in professionalism and, in turn, new forms of trust building that may further participation of service users.

Demanding control and seeking trust: a parallel march

Provision of health care is a societal field in which trust plays a key part at a number of levels. In this context, the significance of trust as a regulatory mechanism between macro and micro-level regulation, and between individuals, organisations and state institutions, comes to the fore. Even if information on health care has improved, the power and knowledge gap between health professionals and service users remains striking (Gilson, 2003), and trust may serve to bridge this gap. However, the trust of citizens and patients in the provision of health care is increasingly challenged. Medical scandals, deficits in the organisation of providers and the quality and efficiency of care on the one hand, and scarcity of resources and the various forms of rationing of health care on the other, are some of the reasons for the eventual erosion of trust in the health care system.

Faced with this situation, all Western states are in the process of introducing new models of governance in order to improve the control of providers and public safety (Allsop and Jones, 2006: forthcoming). As described earlier, in Chapter Two, these developments appear in health systems, firstly, under the catchwords of performance indicators, EBM and quality management (Schepers and Casparie, 1999; Exworthy et al, 2003; Timmermans and Berg, 2003), and are subsumed, in a wider context, as NPM and new governance (Newman, 2001). Secondly, service users are increasingly included in the stakeholder regulation (Baggott et al, 2005; Davies et al, 2005), and, as discriminating and informed consumers (Chapter One, this volume), they are expected to exercise the control of health care providers.

Changes in institutional regulation and health policy are accompanied by changes in the resources and strategies for building trust. Information gleaned from the Internet, for example, and a growing consumer movement have led to a diversification of medical knowledge and increased interest in CAM. Consequently, resources for building trust in health care providers have become more diverse and contradictory. Trust built up in the interactions between professionals and between providers and users is supplemented and extended with assessment and control.

These developments beg the question of whether new managerial regulations simply function as a substitute for trust (Mechanic, 1998). Do they replace models of trust, and displace "trust with various criteria of performance and indicators for review and accounting" (Svensson and Evetts, 2003b, p 9)? Do complex systems of accountability and control themselves damage trust (Evetts, 2006b)? Or do new models of governance also change the underlying cultural rules, the expert systems and concepts of professionalism, thus providing new opportunities for building trust?

Surveys carried out in a number of countries report a decline of trust in social institutions (Delhey and Newton, 2003), and a simultaneous increase in trust in doctors. For example, the British Medical Association reported: "Trust in doctors is at its highest for over twenty years. This is higher than the ratio for any other professional group" (BMA, 2004, p 1). High levels of trust in doctors have also been observed in other surveys and European countries (Braun et al, 2003; Calnan and Sanford, 2004). Accordingly, there is no evidence for an overall decline of trust, nor of its significance in health care. Moreover, we can conclude that a decline in trust in institutions and high levels of trust in doctors coexist. However, this coexistence is characterised by instability. The medical profession simultaneously releases 'traces of doubt' and provides 'sources of trust' (Kuhlmann, 2006b, p 607).

Giddens notes that, "attitudes of trust, as well as more pragmatic acceptance, scepticism, rejection and withdrawal uneasily co-exist in the social sphere linking individual activities and expert systems" (1991, p 7). This 'uneasiness' is currently gaining ground against the backdrop of complex systems of control. Given the importance of trust for the legitimacy of states and the capacity of societies to solve problems, the gap between trust in the macro-level of regulation and trust in individual professionals is troubling. This gap raises two questions: what are the resources and strategies to build trust in the provision of health care, and how are they challenged and changed by new regulatory models?

According to Giddens (1991), trust is based on symbolical signs and expert systems, but not in the sense of the moral principles and good intentions of others. Decisive, above all, is the belief in the soundness of principles of which one knows nothing. Douglas illustrates this connection with respect to radiation therapy, which "has an exceptional tradition of mutual trust and excellent cooperation. Scientists possess accepted methods to verify their claims; they believe in their methods and trust their results in the same way physicians and patients trust one another" (1991, p 14). According to this example, the 'production' of trust is tied to shared values and a common acceptance of methods employed.

With the expert system and scientific methods a direct link is established to the professions and the methods of testing, and thus to the formalised codes of professionalism. The crucial point is that the new models of governance themselves enhance new dynamics in the relationship between trust and contracts in public sector management (Coulson, 1998a) and the symbols of legitimacy and power (Newman, 1998). Negotiations on professionalism are therefore a central component in any model aimed at building trust.

Linking trust and professionalism

When trust is seen as a dynamic rather than a static dimension of professionalism, then new forms of assessment of health care provision and users' calls for informed and self-determined decisions are not necessarily signals of distrust. Rather, such calls can be seen as adaptive measures applied to changed requirements. From this point of view, the first thing we have to decide is no longer whether new models of regulation nurture or hinder trust. Of more interest is how they transform professionalism and how they are used to safeguard its competency and regulatory power.

This theoretical framework opens up further perspectives. First of all, it makes it possible to overcome the concept of 'countervailing powers' of the state, the market and the professions (Mechanic, 1991; Light, 1995; Freidson, 2001), and allows us to analyse negotiation processes and the new arrangements of the actors involved. Secondly, service users – who are viewed only with regard to their market position in the classical triangle of state, market and the professions – can be appropriately taken into account as actors. Thirdly, trust and bureaucratic/managerial regulation are not presented as opposite sides of the scales. On the contrary, this form of regulation becomes a prerequisite for trust under changing requirements.

The regulatory power of trust in health care is directly related to the normative strength of an expert knowledge system, which is ensured by traditional tools of professional self-regulation and embodied in social institutions. These tools are subject to changing patterns of governance aimed at tighter control of providers, and at the same time the desire for seeking trust in medical services continues to exist (Chapter Seven). To better understand the interplay between the paradoxical wishes for seeking trust and demanding control, it is necessary to highlight the coexistence of different dimensions of building trust and the interplay of more stable and new elements of professionalism. According to Allsop and Saks:

> [Trust] may derive in part from the fact that the health professional is defined as the expert and the person seeking help is not, as well as the formal existence of professional ethical and disciplinary codes – however poorly or otherwise these may be implemented in practice. (2002b, p 6)

This statement directs attention to the fact that trust is based on both a 'corporeal order' of professionalism – the expert–lay divide – and a system of formalised codes. Consequently, shifts in one order pattern do not predict similar shifts in the other one. Moreover, there are various options to redefine the existing resources for the building of trust in health care providers and to create new ones. The crucial issue is whether and how symbolic changes interact with changes in professional practice and the regulatory framework of health care. If we take the transformability of professionalism according to new demands on accountability and the ambiguous mix of 'pragmatic acceptance' and 'scepticism' (Giddens, 1991) in citizens' strategies of building trust into account, change in state regulation does not necessarily damage the regulatory power of trust. Moreover, the dynamics of new governance may also enhance new patterns of building trust in professional services.

Regulatory power of trust in the field of health care

From a sociological point of view, Simmel was one of the first to identify trust as the "most important synthetic force in society" (1950, p 326). In recent years numerous authors have taken up this issue, and confirm its growing significance in modernisation processes in society at large (for instance, Coleman, 1990; Giddens, 1991), and changes in public services in particular. Coulson describes trust as the "foundation of public sector management" (1998b, p 3). However, trust is a social category that is not easy to grasp. Power is drawn from its incidence and high relevance within very different social contexts. Trust includes cognitive criteria of decision making as well as subjective dimensions. The latter – which I call 'embodied' – touch on the highly complex nature of individual perceptions, desires and emotions embedded in social conditions of life. Thus, this category lies at odds with the dichotomies of 'private' and 'public', 'experts' and 'lay persons'; it creeps through the mind–body divide, and also crosses the macro and micro-levels of sociological analysis. According to Newman it is the "polyvalence that leads to the problems of talking about trust in a coherent and consistent way" (1998, p 51).

As an interactive category, trust has a considerable influence on the communication between professionals and patients and determines the quality and efficiency of the care provided. The chances for a cure also depend on the level of trust patients place in the medical system and the treatment they receive from physicians (Mechanic and Meyer, 2000). With the growing complexity of medical treatments and therapies, as well as their uncertainties and risks, the importance of and need for trust has increased. The patients in my study highlighted the need for trustworthy relations with health providers. In general, they expressed trust in 'their' doctor. Although they were aware of the deficits of doctors' advice and medical competencies and felt that control of physicians is necessary, they developed a number of tactics to avoid any signs of mistrust in the patient–physician interaction.

It is interesting to note that physicians are the most important source of trust. The patients in my study valued information given by a physician more than information from other health professions and occupations. For example, patients criticised physicians' lack of qualifications and competencies in nutrition and dietary advice, but considered advice from specially trained dietary assistants to be less trustworthy than that given by physicians (Chapter Seven). These results mirror the physician-centred structure of the German health system and low degree of user trust in health occupations compared to physicians (Braun et al, 2003). Physicians in my study also emphasised the significance of trust as an important condition of high-quality care. They felt a need to win back trust in their services. To a certain degree professional identities and agency are based on the levels of trust patients and the public bring to these services and the willingness of physicians to act according to an altruistic ethos as advocates of patients (Chapter Five).

The relationship between trust and health care seems to be most crucial on the interactive level of the patient–physician relationship (Thiede, 2005). Its importance and regulatory power, however, goes far beyond this. Trust is not only related to professional identities as moral conduct (Hellberg, 1999), it can also generate impulses that lead to structural changes. The capacity of trustworthy relations between physicians to enhance change is clearly borne out by the improvement of cooperation, coordination and teamwork in health care. Results of my study confirm that the advance of networks and quality circles of physicians and also improved cooperation with health occupations are especially enhanced by trust. The wish for trustworthy relations and individual support was an important motive for physicians to establish or join networks (Chapter Six).

Economic considerations of trust also become apparent at this level (Gilson, 2003). Nurturing a culture of trust at the organisational level can optimise the efficiency of the providers and their working methods. The quality circles of German physicians bring this dimension of trust into view; quality of care can be improved through an environment of trustworthy relations, where physicians learn to report on problems and deficits. They hereby develop new strategies of problem solving and quality management that may contribute to the efficiency of health care systems (Chapter Six).

The medical profession makes use of trust at various levels. The incentives to win back trust of the public and governments can be viewed as an interest-based strategy to ensure and expand power on the macro-level of regulation. Here, the link between professional interests and states comes to the fore. In the end, the legitimacy of a government is derived to no small degree from citizens' trust in the health care it provides. The medical profession plays a pivotal role, positioned as it is between the interests of the state and citizens as beneficiaries of health care (Harrison and Ahmad, 2000). A comparative study of the German, Austrian, British and Danish health systems reveals that neither the biggest budgets and number of staff nor the degree of freedom of choice for users are positively correlated with high levels of trust and satisfaction of users. According to data from the Eurobarometer, the Danish health system ranked first, despite cuts made in health care expenditure since the 1980s (Wendt, 2003, p 389). The results lead us back to the question of the resources for building trust. Gilson identifies five areas, which are influenced by trust:

> [Trust] builds relationships that underlie economic development; builds legitimacy of governance institutions, may promote ethical outcomes in society; builds legitimacy and so capacity of public systems; employee trust in employer enhances morale and motivation, and so organisational performance; reduces the need to monitor and so reduces transaction costs and enhances ability to manage complexity. (2003, p 1455)

Changes in the governance of health care may play out differently in the various areas of building trust; the challenge is to grasp the dynamic relationship between new patterns of governance and the medical professions' room for manoeuvre to mobilise new resources of building trust in doctors.

New models of governance and the building of trust

New models of governance directly impact on the building of trust, but in various ways. Studies carried out in the US concentrate on the country's MCOs and emphasise, for the main part, their negative influences on trustworthy relations. For example, Mechanic argues that "patients continue to express high confidence in their personal physicians but changes in employer health insurance decisions and increasing market penetration of HMOs are disrupting many existing relationships and eroding patient trust" (1998, p 662; see Ahern and Hendryx, 2003; Thom et al, 2004). From this perspective it is the relationship between "public trust and physicians' agency" (Mechanic, 1998, p 669) that is being addressed. Mechanic focuses on the organisational arrangements and the interpersonal skills' capacity to elicit trust in medicine and emphasises the spillover effects in both directions. He does not, however, analyse what new forms of professionalism these spillover effects can give rise to and what possibilities they, in turn, create for building trust.

Harrison and Smith (2004) also argue the thesis of decline of trust in societies from a British perspective, but go further than identifying negative effects on trust simply from certain policies and organisational changes. The authors put changing patterns of regulation in health care in the context of modernisation processes, and explore four elements in relation to trust: 'surveillance' (inspection, monitoring and evaluating performance), 'bureaucracy' (governing performance with rules and procedures), 'instrumentality' (evidence-based practice) and 'consumerism' (empowering service users). Following their argument these elements of policy imperatives bear the mark of modernisation and thus raise a similar problem: "the modernisation agenda privileges confidence over trust and neglects the relationship between trust, moral motivation and uncertainty. This has important consequences for service providers and service users" (2004, p 375). The authors view confidence, positioned at the centre of policy initiatives, and trust, positioned at the periphery, as opposite ends of the scale. The problem of the concept of trust developed by Harrison and Smith is that it links policies and 'frontline' interactions between providers and service users to a single organising order of modernity.

However, empirical data point to uneven developments. Surveys in three European countries – Germany, the Netherlands and England/ Wales – reveal that there is no evidence that trust and confidence in health care in general are in decline, although the public now seems to be more critical about medical treatment and expert advice (Braun et al, 2003). Despite many differences in the trust in health care expressed in each of these countries, trust in physicians is generally very high – between 80% and 90%. However, trust in communication competencies and the information given by physicians ranks much lower (40% to 60%) (Braun et al, 2003, p 155). The similarities between the three nations are not confirmed with regard to trust in the various health professions and providers of alternative medicine. For example, trust in nurses and physiotherapists is highest in England and Wales –

and equal to trust in specialised physicians – and about 20% higher than in Germany.

Even more striking, however, are the differences in the area of CAM. While roughly 87% of citizens in England and Wales expressed trust in alternative medicine provided by physicians, the comparable figure is only 42% in Germany. Similarly, alternative healers are trusted by about 57% in England and Wales but by just 12% in Germany (Braun et al, 2003, p 150). The authors conclude that the relationship between organisational, material and political changes in health care and the building of trust is weaker than assumed, and that additional research and categories are needed to highlight the complex relationship.

Additional analysis was undertaken for the German survey data (Braun and Schnee, 2002). The authors show that more than 80% of the patients surveyed expressed trust in generalists, specialists and dentists. With respect to the resources of building trust, the data reveal paradoxes. Notably, about 30% had changed their physician at least once, often because of disagreement about therapy (Braun and Schnee, 2002, p 179), and 69% called for more information about the quality of physicians and hospitals (Marstedt, 2003, p 119). A more detailed analysis of the reasons for using multiple sources to gather information beyond physicians' advice highlights that the desire for information is not correlated to communication deficits in the patient–physician interaction or dissatisfaction with this information (Marstedt, 2003, p 126).

Following the author's interpretation the search for information marks social and cultural changes of the role of patients in health care, which allows for more active citizens' participation and personal engagement in decision making (Marstedt, 2003, p 135). Qualitative material from my study underscores this interpretation. Patients perceived information from different sources as an important condition of self-determined decisions and emphasised a positive impact on the building of trust in their own doctor (Chapter Seven). These changes bring into focus new implications for information, and new demands on professionalism and professional competencies.

Building trust through 'visible markers'

In times of new governance, building trust in health care remains vital, but the medical profession has to justify the placing of trust and compete for it with other experts; competition takes place even within the profession. Data show that physicians' qualifications and the traditional biomedical expert system – while still important – no longer guarantee a sufficient basis for trust building. Notably, physicians and patients search for proof and signifiers of trustworthiness (Chapters Six and Seven). In this situation, new concepts of professionalism are emerging that integrate tools from quality management. As described in Chapter Six, professionalism and managerialism are increasingly merging. These changes in the meaning of professionalism induce complex processes of change, in which resources for building trust are developed. Physicians often perceive managerial regulation as external control and loss of self-determination. However, my findings indicate that these tools are also used to strengthen the position of the medical profession at meso and macro-levels. Similar conclusions were drawn from changes in the British health system:

> At these levels there is an increased reliance on medical expertise rather than a diminution of medical influence and authority.[...] Doctors still own expertise in all the areas where regulation has grown; regulators, from judges to managers, invariably rely on an expert input to their decision making. (Allsop, 1999, pp 168-9; see Harrison and Ahmad, 2000)

According to these results, trust in expert knowledge is increasing rather than declining. At the meso-level new tools offer the medical profession possibilities of mutual assessment. Used in this way trustful cooperation between physicians can be strengthened, as described by physicians working in networks, and professional power can be ensured (Chapter Six).

Patient data (Chapter Seven) make it apparent that trust in the provider of general care and the wish for additional information from a specialist and from a seemingly neutral resource, such as the media, the Internet or a patient information centre, are complementary, and not perceived as a contradiction. Moreover, patients build trust in 'their' doctor, even if they perceive his or her knowledge to be limited and go on to seek additional advice and information from other sources. Many patients in my study reported bad experiences – which in part seriously damaged the health of patients and reduced their chances of good care – and disappointment with medical treatment. It was also reported that the information given by physicians is not always up to date, and does not cover the entire spectrum of what patients want to know about treatment options.

Despite the awareness of many deficits, however, patients generally trust 'their' doctor. They feel themselves capable of finding the 'right' physician, who will provide 'good' care. This confidence in their own judgement and ability to make informed decisions is related to the increased access people have to diverse sources of information. The possibility to make decisions based on 'rational' criteria is perceived as a prerequisite for building trust and for taking a more active role in decision making.

The new instruments of assessment offer service users a way to judge for themselves the provision of the health professions and organisations beyond their own subjective experiences. Trust, previously founded on a more or less 'embodied' basis, is supplemented with 'rational' evaluation criteria, like the performance indicators. Here too we ascertain that diminishing trust in health care systems goes hand in hand with new trust-building measures at the micro-level, which make a more active role possible for patients in their interactions with physicians. As Thiede recently wrote: "information may enlarge individual choice sets and increase the freedom to use health care; it serves as a stimulus to access" (2005, p 1452). In addition, on the macro and meso-levels user representatives are increasingly involved in the decision processes that deal with the definition of quality and effectiveness of health services. Although involvement might still be weak, citizenship rights and participation are leading to improvements. On a symbolic level the active involvement of user representatives in the health policy process challenges the 'corporeal order' based on a strong expert–lay divide. New resources of building trust are thus made available on the macro-level of regulation that can be employed to enhance trust at the micro-level of patient–physician interaction.

Taking up on Douglas (1991), we can say that, in addition to the pluralisation of resources for trust, more complex test methods have to be renegotiated and this will mean changes in the demands on and expectations of professionalism. However, to view this development only under the aspect of growing mistrust falls short of reality. New managerial instruments can be employed by the different actors and may thus help to build trust at many different levels. In a quantitative dimension it is hardly possible to predict yet whether trust will rise or fall. Of more importance is the question that addresses the qualitative changes in building trust. What will replace the paternalistic authority of the physician and bridge the gap between expert and lay perspectives? This question leads to the issue of information and its potential for changing the asymmetrical relations in health care.

Information: the bridge between trust and control

If ever more actors are included in decision-making processes, and resources for building trust become ever more diverse, demand rises for regulation and negotiation between different actors and cultural value systems. Information takes on a new meaning within this context. Webster points out that, "the arrival of the 'expert patient' simply gives a further twist to the technical ratchet", and concludes that "the demand for visible markers justifying experts' decisions is likely to grow" (2002, p 451). At present this call for visible markers is fulfilled by scientific-bureaucratic regulation via tools from the realms of management. Physicians, patients, insurance companies and health policy makers all rely on EBM, quality management, data from evaluations, audits and documentation of health care services. However, the regulatory power is not derived solely from the broad acceptance of the tools themselves, but from the shared belief in the information they carry.

Information is often viewed as a tool of market governance that creates conflict between service providers and users. As a metaphor, however, information has the potential to serve different actors and demands; it amalgamates the call for control and the desire for trust. Information is the 'bridge' between the various players in health care and between doubt and trust. It is the core of a new technology of building trust. In these processes, trust in individuals and embodied practices shifts to trust in neutralised data detached from the body. These shifts appear, for example, in the 'disembodied' physician–patient relationship manifest in telephone counselling, information from the Internet, or medical magazines on television or radio or in print. And video films are sometimes used to rationalise the disclosure of medical diagnosis, which is a key area of personal patient–physician interaction. Shifts towards trust in 'neutralised' data also appear with respect to patients. For example, trust in bodily perceptions is disrupted if feeling healthy depends on what biomedical tests say about the probability of getting ill (Kuhlmann, 2002; Webster, 2002).

As a discourse, information fits very well with other familiar discourses on 'network society', 'individualisation' and 'risk society' in that it promises self-determined decision making and participation. It seems to bridge the power gap between experts and lay people. Information does not always have to prove its worth, it becomes a new 'signifier' of quality of care and also of 'freedom of choice' and participation of citizens. These developments have mainly been studied for new areas of biotechnology and human genetics, where analysis focuses on the aspect of the technicalisation of medicine. As a symbolic sign of modernisation, however, information is spreading over the entire area of health care.

Increased information leads to vociferous calls for the control of opaque and sometimes risky medical treatments and therapies, as well as patients' demands for more self-determination. Results show that physicians take up this call and improve the information for patients (Chapter Five, this volume). Shared decision making and informed consent is a qualitatively new dimension in the relationship between physician and patient, and it is achieved for the main part via information. Increasingly, justified trust in health care is founded on information, and the 'carriers' are the tools from the realms of NPM. That this development is ambivalent and entails no little amount of risk, that it marginalises emotional, 'felt' forms of building trust, and furthers the individualisation of responsibility for health, has been discussed elsewhere (Kuhlmann, 2002). Here, I wish to emphasise the redefinition of trust and the effects on the power structure of health care.

Information does not automatically abolish asymmetries in health systems (Lee and Garvin, 2003). The empirical data discussed in Chapter Seven confirm, firstly, that information and disclosure are governed by what physicians deem to be relevant for patients, and, secondly, that the effective use of information depends on the underlying expert system and its normative power. I will return to the latter issue in the next chapter. Furthermore, the growing significance of information produces new social inequalities in health and access to health care services. The patients in my study give several examples that access to information is related to social status and 'cultural capital'. Freedom of choice is thus the freedom of healthy and wealthy citizens rather than the poor and sick. Nonetheless, on the symbolical level the information metaphor also embodies potential for changes within the medical profession and between physicians, patients and the public.

With respect to this issue, Sarasin's historical analysis of the making of a new medical discourse offers comprehensive insights with which to gauge the consequences of the changes underway. Sarasin asks whether – and if so, why – the authority of scientific, especially medical, knowledge will remain intact "when not this or that renowned professor, but an unknown physician in a cheap brochure or in the advice column of a magazine" is the source of information (2001, p 141). The issue is addressed and developed using the example of the discourse on hygiene at the end of the 19th century. The author raises the question as to whether we can "find anything in the discourse on hygiene that backed up the physician and lent authority to his words?" (2001, p 141). According to Sarasin, trust is not merely built up in individual physician–patient relationships but is based on a symbolical order that is represented by the physician:

> Natural laws successfully competed with God's laws in the middle of the 19th century and associated themselves with the new political and equally quasi-transcendental models of nation states, and were presented to enlightened subjects as the reason for their societal existence. This law is a guarantee of a world and corporeal order, personified by physicians and scientists. The authors advocate not only the placing of trust in physicians – the sick more or less never had a real choice – but trust in that concrete physical law that determines the 'chemical–physical experiment' of one's own life. (Sarasin, 2001, p 146)

Sarasin's analysis reminds us that trust in health care is not only tied to paternalism but also to a gendered expert system that privileges the interests of men. He argues that the personification of this natural law is "the father figure of the scholar, whose name guarantees that the uninitiated submit to the symbolical" (2001, p 146). When these personalised and embodied signifiers of trust are now replaced with disembodied ones, which are based, moreover, on transparency and 'rational' criteria, there are very good reasons not to regret the changes under way but to seek out and embrace the chances they offer.

Redefining trust: modernising professionalism

The traditional form of building trust via the physician acting as an agent for the patient is undergoing redefinition. Calls are increasing for visible markers of trust, and the new tools of bureaucratic regulation and performance indicators fulfil this function as signifiers of quality. They are taken up by the medical profession and integrated into their individual professional practices as well as professional politics (Chapter Five, this volume). Patients also refer to the new signifiers of quality. As a result, a number of fissures and breaks appear in the heroic image of doctors who rescue humankind from illness and rule over health and health care systems. This is true for both the professional identity of physicians (Chapter Six, this volume) as well as for the views of patients on the limited knowledge and competencies of physicians (Chapter Seven, this volume).

In this context new patterns of medical governance do not merely provide new tools, but are rather the expression of a new technology of building trust via information under conditions of uncertainty and a 'risk society' (Beck, 1986). These processes can be seen in a broader context of societal change and modernisation processes, which is discussed under the headings of individualisation, self-determination and citizenship. From a sociological point of view, the really interesting change does not lie in the instruments themselves, but in the transformation of the symbols and the effects of this in the area of health care. The technology of building trust on visible markers and justifiable criteria mirrors the superstructure of citizenship that governs the transformation of welfare states (Chapter One, this volume).

This technology perfectly fits the image of 'reflexive actors' and 'expert patients' who exercise control over providers, as well as the discretionary decision making of 'autonomous' professionals. It has the capacity to bridge new demands on social inclusion and participation on the one hand, and classical values and claims of professions on the other. Findings indicate that new strategies of building trust contribute to the expansion of professionalism, and serve well the regulation of social relations under conditions of complexity and uncertainty on macro, meso and micro-levels. The flexibility and transformability of professionalism allows for the inclusion of new demands without necessarily weakening professional power. Proof of the trustworthiness of the health professionals is still founded on expert systems; and physicians and biomedical knowledge, especially in Germany, rank first in trustworthiness by the public.

At the same time, the shifts in professionalism towards information and 'rational' criteria for trustworthiness also embody potential for reducing hierarchy in health care. Dynamics are enhanced on different levels: the expert–lay divide, gender relations and the system of health professions and occupations. A classic pattern of professionalism is traditionally linked to a male body and serves – most of the time – the interests of white, upper or middle-class male actors. When trust in professionals becomes more detached from the body and is increasingly founded in disembodied signifiers, it can be conjectured that the changes may open up new participation chances for female health professionals. For example, a classic gendered pattern of low user trust in technical and surgical competencies of female physicians has disappeared in some countries (Kerssens et al, 1997; Chapter Two, this volume). These developments may help to reduce gender hierarchy in the health workforce.

In this respect, the higher scores of trustworthiness achieved by

English and Dutch compared to German nurses and physiotherapists (Braun et al, 2003) need to be investigated more fully to assess the relationship between quality assessment and trust, as medical governance is more advanced and the regulation more open to user participation in England (Allsop et al, 2002; Davies et al, 2005) and the Netherlands (Kremer, 2005). Results so far reveal a complex and hardly predictable interplay of citizens' trust in providers, improved user power and shifts in the (gendered) division of labour in health care.

The crucial point is that shifts on different levels may intersect in various ways. This interplay may enhance new tensions and dynamics that, in turn, may reduce the existing power gaps in health care but also produce new social inequalities. For example, an unequal distribution of access to and use of information between social groups of users produces new social inequalities (Chapter Seven, this volume). And unequal access of the medical and the allied health professions and occupations to the recourses of legitimising information via scientific evidence – as described, for instance, with respect to German physiotherapists (Chapter Six, this volume) – may reinforce the division of labour or produce new divisions. Accordingly, the relationship between new regulatory tools and the options to build trust must be assessed in context (Goudge and Gilson, 2005). According to Newman, "techniques alone will not succeed unless they are accompanied by a transformation of the institution itself" (1998, p 49). This leads us from the shifts in the symbols and discourse back to changes in the institutions and structure of health care.

Remodelling medical governance

Coming back to the significance of trust and its linkage to professionalism and governance we can conclude that social effects and dynamics cannot be assessed on any one level of change but must be set in a broader context of modernisation processes in society. The 'embodied' dimension of trust and its mediation via physicians remains crucial but is increasingly related to 'rational' criteria and proof of trustworthiness. Despite the ambivalences of these transformations, new forms of professionalism emerge that open pathways for negotiations and rearrangements of the existing power relations in health care.

New governance and complex systems of control of physicians do not necessarily damage the power of the medical profession and the capacity of professions to build trust and solve the problems of the society. As described earlier, in Chapter Five, physicians are not simply the 'objects' of new governance but actively take up and remodel new patterns of regulation. The medical profession makes use of new signifiers of trust provided by tools from medical governance. Physicians supplement classical 'embodied' signifiers of building trust with new signifiers based on information, thus successfully ensuring trust in their services under changing requirements. On the macro-level of regulation, however, the symbolic power of 'embodied' signifiers of trust is weaker than on the interactive level, and, as a consequence, there are fewer trust-building resources. Shifting the resources of trustworthy relations towards 'rational' criteria of evaluation may therefore impact on macro and micro-levels of health care in different ways and affect the players involved in different ways. While tools from new governance may serve as public proof of the trustworthiness of physicians, they may also damage the building of trust in the government and its institutions.

A gap between trust in doctors and trust in social institutions is observed in different health care systems (Braun et al, 2003; Wendt, 2003). One of the reasons for this gap may be a result of various ways of amalgamating the components of trust described by Giddens (1991) in different social contexts with different requirements. On the micro-level of interaction the 'pragmatic acceptance' may gain greater significance than 'scepticism' and 'withdrawal'. Often, patients have no real 'choice' and cannot reject a doctor's advice in the face of an urgent need for help. Compared with this situation, there is no direct dependency and urgent call for decision making when it comes to judgements on health policy and state regulation, and here more sceptical components may dominate the pattern of building trust.

In this situation, professionals can serve as mediators between different social areas and patterns of building trust. A high degree of involvement of the professions at the macro-level of regulation and strong patterns of self-regulation may result in further spillover effects from micro-levels of interaction into the area of policy decisions, and extend resources for building trust in governments. Following this argument the positioning of professions in the regulatory arrangement is an essential issue for the levels of trust that citizens have in their governments. Subsequently, shifts in the balance of power may enhance shifts in citizens' trust in governments.

In Germany, the corporatist arrangement is based on a partial delegation of the state's power and responsibility to the medical profession and the SHI funds. Under these conditions the call for tighter control of providers might turn out to be a boomerang for the state rather than a threat to medical power. It brings into question the whole system of regulation, and subsequently, the legitimacy and capacity of the state to serve the interests of its citizens. These potentially adverse effects of new models of governance were observed with respect to patients' demands on health care (Chapter Seven, this volume). Patients take up the new promises of participation and citizenship rights. They do not, however, accept a mere shift from the medical profession towards the SHI funds but address their demands directly to the government, for example by calling for health policies that provide better and safer information on health care providers.

The spotlight has been turned on the deficits of the current pattern of corporatism in Germany: while health policy attempts to better control physicians and reduce medical power, it may damage the role of the medical profession as mediator between state and citizens and a 'stabiliser' of governance, thus reducing trust-building sources. First, negative effects are especially strong because state regulation is weak, the move towards tighter control slow and the tools incomplete. Second, the regulatory arrangement fails to ensure the inclusion of new actors, such as users and health occupations, although changes are under way with respect to service users. Accordingly, regulatory shifts towards tighter control of the medical profession and its power to target developments in health care mean that changes need to be made in the institutions and regulatory system itself to include new actors.

NINE

The knowledge–power knot in professionalism: transforming the 'currency of competition'

Knowledge is the key to professional power and the 'currency of competition' in the service sector. New models of governance that attempt to standardise knowledge and include user perspectives thus touch the core of professional power. This chapter contextualises the making of legitimate knowledge and outlines the conditions and options for a loosening of the knowledge–power knot of professionalism. I introduce a dynamic approach that moves beyond state control and market regulation, and links the approaches on knowledge and professionalism as a resource for occupational control with the social construction of knowledge. The findings of the study highlight that the new models of standardising and monitoring knowledge challenge – but do not necessarily threaten – professional power. Moreover, they open up new options for the medical profession to legitimise knowledge and power, and hereby challenge health policies that attempt to improve the control of providers. Bringing together different approaches and empirical findings reveals evidence of a diversity of knowledge and a more empowering potential of standardisation, but also of an increasing 'rationalisation' that serves to reassure medical power under changing conditions of marketisation and consumerism.

Challenging the alliance of knowledge, power and professionalism

A body of esoteric knowledge and a formalised expert knowledge system are key issues in studying the professions (Parsons, 1949; Freidson, 1986; Thorstendahl and Burrage, 1990). However, new forms of regulating the health professions and 'managing' the making of legitimate knowledge necessitate further investigation of the alliance between knowledge and professional power. Linking the approaches on knowledge as a resource for occupational control with the social construction and feminist theorising of knowledge, provides deeper insights into the ambivalence of formalised codes of knowledge and the tensions between professions, the state and the public.

Current changes provoked by consumerism and 'scientific-bureaucratic medicine' (Harrison, 1998) are key issues to assess the power and transformability of professional knowledge. Flynn argues that "the intermediate concepts of soft bureaucracy and encoded knowledge" are useful to understand the nature of organisational control in health care (2004, p 24). However, my empirical findings indicate that these concepts must be linked to the actors who apply and transform the new regulatory tools in different ways, as well as to the institutional contexts that shape these options.

The new models of regulating the health professions and occupations are governed by the assumption that the standardisation of knowledge and the inclusion of new actors in the negotiation processes will improve both the accountability of professions and citizenship rights (Chapter Two, this volume). Unwarranted practice variations of provider services and interest-based strategies of the professions are to be reduced through clearly defined standards of care, formalised codes – such as EBM and decision making – and clinical guidelines. Performance indicators target the provision of care; the process and outcome are more closely monitored and controlled by evaluations and audits. Tools from NPM serve as drivers for modernisation processes (Chapter Four, this volume) and provide 'public proof' of the accountability of professions and the quality of care.

The inclusion of lay knowledge of users generates further changes in the knowledge system and challenges the supremacy of medical knowledge. New patterns of governing the professions promise new opportunities to loosen the knowledge–power knot (Clarke et al, 2005). Newman and Vidler highlight that, although challenges on clinical autonomy through marketisation and managerialism are not new, "for the first time the service user comes to embody the challenge" (2006: forthcoming). Knowledge has thus come under scrutiny from different sides. However, the 'parallel march' of scientific-bureaucratic medicine and consumerism needs a critical review to assess the social effects on the system of health care and the power relations in this arena.

Controversy continues concerning the democratic potential of standardisation and the pathways open to new 'knowers' and knowledge systems. Cognitive standardisation is a classic strategy of professions to gain occupational closure and dominance over other groups. However, this strategy co-exists with the 'tacit knowledge' and discretionary decision making of professionals. The 'mystic' of expert knowledge, as Turner (1995) calls it, can also be used as a barrier against external regulation. Accordingly, new health policies that shift the balance towards standardisation of knowledge do not necessarily transform the exclusionary tactics and demarcation processes of the professions into more inclusive patterns of professionalism. Moreover, the professions can flexibly utilise and balance different strategies – formalised and 'tacit' knowledge – to ensure power. Professional knowledge thus poses a dual challenge to public control, and provides various options to counteract tighter control.

In contrast to this, new health policies are underpinned by the assumption that managing professional knowledge translates in a linear sequence into frontline changes in health care. This logic, however, borrowed from management and the economy, underestimates the power of the medical profession to construct and make use of standardisation, to include new knowledge claims and to transform its knowledge base according to new demands. It also neglects the mediating role of the professions in health care and the normative power of the biomedical knowledge system in society at large (Chapter Seven). There is hardly another area of knowledge in which the expert system is held in such high esteem as in biomedicine.

Taking the reflexivity and transformability of professionalism into account leads us from a rather static concept of knowledge and power based on the assumption of conflicting logic between professions and the service users towards a more dynamic approach, which highlights the processes rather than the tools used to make legitimate knowledge. This allows us to focus on the interactions and tensions between the interests of the different players involved in these processes. The crucial issue is whether new actors are involved in the negotiations on standards and criteria of quality of care, and how the government targets the inclusion of new 'knowers' in the production of knowledge. The question up for discussion is whether the transformation of knowledge enhanced through patterns of new governance follows the pathway of unique truth claims as an essential feature of modernity (Haraway, 1997), or whether it is capable of developing a social order of knowledge that contributes to diversity and participation in accordance with the changing modes of citizenship. These questions are addressed in the following sections.

Knowledge and power: moving beyond standardisation and mystic

Numerous authors have studied the tensions between knowledge and professionalism using different theoretical approaches. A major part of the body of the literature deals with knowledge and a formalised system as a resource for professional power that is used to gain occupational closure and dominance over other groups. Freidson (1986) is one of the prominent writers in this area. In recent work he has developed an ideal-type of professional knowledge "as a kind of specialization considered to be both discretionary and based on abstract concepts and theories" (2001, p 152). This model stands as 'third logic' next to those of rational-legal bureaucracy developed by Max Weber, which represents managerialism, and "Adam Smith's model of the free market which represents consumerism" (Freidson, 2001, p 179).

The importance of abstraction of knowledge, "effective enough to compete in a particular historical and social context", is confirmed in the work of Abbott (1988, p 9) and Larson (1977). Both authors emphasise the process character of the social construction of expertise. While Abbott focuses on the jurisdiction of work, Larson outlines the rationalisation and standardisation of knowledge as exclusionary strategies to secure market power. She highlights the power of cognitive standardisation as the generator of deeply shared cultural assumptions. Of most interest to the questions under discussion, she brings the "dialectics between indetermination and codification" into focus (1977, p 41):

> Both historically and logically, standardization appears to have a democratic potential: because it reduces the margins of indetermination and secrecy, standardization broadens the possibilities of access to a body of technical and cognitive skills. It tends, therefore, to be advocated by those who are excluded from the occupational privileges based on secrecy. (Larson, 1977, p 42)

Turner (1995) further outlined the notion of ambivalence. Like Larson, he refers to the historical study of the medical profession in France by Jamous and Pelloille, and argues that the knowledge of professions "has to have a distinct mystique which suggests that there is a certain professional attitude and competence that cannot be reduced merely to systematic and routinized knowledge" (1995, p 133). According to Turner it is this mystic that provides the barrier against external control and regulation.

Following this argument, the ongoing standardisation of knowledge currently under way in scientific-bureaucratic medicine and health policy is perceived as a threat to professional power and as bringing new opportunities to improve participation of 'outsiders', such as users and the various allied health professions and occupations. Accordingly, classic approaches from the sociology of professions mirror the logic of health policies and vice versa. However, empirical findings do not fully confirm these assumptions but reveal that the medical profession is capable, at least in part, of counteracting policy aims. As described in Chapter Six, physicians successfully translate the tools of standardising knowledge into an interest-based strategy of professionalisation.

In her later work, Larson seems to be more sceptical regarding the democratic potential of standardisation: "The boundary that protects cognitive fields towards the outside [...] means that only the knowers themselves will define what are valid subjects of knowledge and valid criteria of pertinence and truth" (1990, p 31). This approach directs attention to the players who sit at the table when standards are negotiated. It remains weak, however, when it comes to the connections between the 'outsiders' and the 'knowers' and the processes of 'making' legitimate knowledge.

Making of legitimate knowledge

The link between power and knowledge based on formalised codes and rationalised technique is a key issue in the work of Foucault (1979) and his concept of governmentality (Dean, 1999). Several writers take this concept on board and focus on the capacity of knowledge technologies, via audits and suchlike, to govern at a distance and assess the activities of experts (for instance, Rose, 1999). Johnson (1995) brings the strategic role of professions into view. He proposes to overcome the rather static and contradictory conception of external regulation and professionalism:

> In short, the state, as the particular form that government has taken in the modern world, includes expertise, or the professions. [...] the 'neutrality' of professional expertise, where it exists, is itself an outcome of a political process rather than the product of some inherent essence, such as esoteric knowledge. (1995, pp 12-13, 18)

This statement points to an important dimension of professional knowledge, namely its claim to possess neutrality, objectivity and universalism. This "heroic journey of mastery of knowledge", as Davies puts it (2002a, p 99), fits well with the criteria of the new scientific-bureaucratic medicine; here, the "production of objectivity" (Timmermans and Berg, 2003, p 117) plays a major role.

The mechanisms and processes of making knowledge and the underlying social order of hierarchy and inequality are most clearly outlined by feminist authors, and also emphasised in the field of so-called post-structural and social construction theorising. Claims for universalism and relativism are identified as the "conquering gaze" that "signifies the unmarked positions of Man and White" (Haraway, 1991, p 188). They create a detached and deeply self-reliant notion of self as apart from others (Davies, 2002a). The aim of these approaches is to dismantle an ongoing naturalising discourse that "continues to justify 'social' orders in terms of 'natural' legitimations" (Haraway, 1997, p 108). The most important lesson from feminist research and social construction approaches is that power is not inherent in knowledge, but socially constructed and context dependent (Latour and Woolgar, 1986; Mclaughlin and Webster, 1998). However, these approaches do not sufficiently explain how the social construction of knowledge is translated to hierarchy and control in the occupational field, and which dynamics these transformations enhance.

Fournier links these two dimensions of "constitution of the professional field [...] and the making of this independent field into a legitimate area of knowledge of and intervention on the world" (2000, p 69):

> Seeing professional knowledge and the constitution of this field as performative and malleable, as an achievement [...] rather than a discovery and reflection of the 'true nature' of some independent reality, suggests the possibility for the professions to reconstitute their field and knowledge in line with the version(s) of reality popularised by recent discourses celebrating the value of the market and enterprise. (2000, p 83)

The author reminds us of the "power of professional knowledge to remake itself, to reconstruct its boundaries" (2000, p 84), and that some professions are better equipped than others to do so.

The processes of defining legitimate knowledge and transforming it into control over another occupational field can be most clearly observed in contested areas of knowledge claims, such as medical genetics (Kuhlmann, 2002), health prevention and promotion (Beattie, 1991) and CAM (Kelner et al, 2004). Research confirms a high flexibility of biomedical knowledge and its 'elastic' potential to include new demands and knowledge systems. With respect to alternative medicine, Saks points out that "it is not always the non-medically qualified who are the standard-bearers for alternative therapies" (2003b, p 163), but often the medical profession itself (Chapter One, this volume).

Research into CAM also gives examples of successful transformations of knowledge claims to new professional projects and identities raised at the margins of health care services (Saks, 1999; Tovey et al, 2004). It is thus not exclusively the 'knowers' who define the expert knowledge system, as Larson (1990) assumed. The knowledge system is also, at least in part, open to 'outsiders' who become 'new knowers', thereby enhancing rearrangements within the power structure. From a historical perspective, medical power over the definition of health and illness and standards of care were inadequate to grasp the entire spectrum; diversity of knowledge was the norm rather than the exception it may appear to have been today (Sharma, 2003).

A further area of transformation in the knowledge basis of professions is gender research. Numerous studies highlight a gender bias in medical knowledge and biomedical theories on health, illness and the body (for instance, Bendelow et al, 2002; Kuhlmann and Babitsch, 2002; Annandale, 2005). In the past, women – together with minority ethnic groups – have been generally excluded from the 'production' of knowledge; as patients, until recently, they were excluded or not adequately included in clinical trials (Healy, 1991); as professionals and citizens they are still in a minority on the boards and in the institutions that define the evidence of medical studies and set the standards of care. In addition, the so-called female professions are either not included in the stakeholder regulation – as described for Germany with respect to physiotherapy (Chapters Three and Five, this volume) – or not acknowledged as equal stakeholders, as borne out, for example, by studies on the regulation of the nursing profession in Britain (Davies, 2002a, 2002b).

A growing body of research on gender differences in health care, together with women's claims for participation, highlight these deficiencies and their negative impact on the quality of care. Accordingly, international organisations have introduced gender-mainstreaming policies (WHO Euro, 2001) and some countries, in particular the US, have set up new regulatory bodies to monitor gender equality in health care (McKinley et al, 2001). These efforts are closely linked to new models of medical governance and tools borrowed from NPM. In this way, the production of knowledge is controlled for gender issues, and biomedical knowledge is complemented with social dimensions of health. Claims of neutrality and objectivity of medical knowledge are challenged when the 'conquering gaze' (Haraway, 1991) of hegemonic masculinity and interest-based strategies of male actors are subjected to public scrutiny, and gender assessment enters the debate on health care and quality. In the same vein, the biomedical gaze is relaxed when consumers are included in the regulatory bodies and demand other than biomedical standards of care, including holistic approaches and alternative therapies (Chapter Seven, this volume).

Transformability of knowledge

The examples on gender research and CAM highlight that knowledge claims are a specific strategy of interest-related claims raised by different groups. The main lesson we can draw from this research is that medical knowledge is highly transformable and not the immovable monolith it is often portrayed as being. There is no guarantee, however, that a mere plurality of knowledge contributes to the diversity of needs and interests in health care. This is equally true for the inclusion of CAM in the health care system as well as for the calls for gender equality. In part, the medical profession takes up these calls and adapts the content and aims of new approaches to meet its own interests. Subsequently, the changes under way do not necessarily provoke sustainable changes in the power relationship, but they do have an initial impact on ongoing negotiations concerning knowledge that may further social inclusion and diversity.

Bringing together the different approaches and findings on knowledge and power reveals that medical knowledge is not just a powerful resource and a masquerade for professional dominance, but a 'creeper' that crosses boundaries. It is capable of shaping and reshaping social structure, culture and action and even individual 'feelings' and agency (Martin, 1994). The patients in my focus groups gave several examples illustrating that a preference for alternative treatments does not necessarily empower patients to reject the definitions of biomedicine in certain situations (Chapter Seven, this volume). Changes in the power of knowledge are thus the outcome of highly complex and ambivalent social processes, which cannot be assessed accurately in a linear formation. Neither the shifts between formalisation and 'mystic' nor the plurality of actors and knowledge systems necessarily weaken the power of biomedical knowledge.

Following the "fluidity of boundaries" argument (Saks, 2003b, p 161) and a "performative and malleable" professionalism (Fournier, 2000, p 83), the transformation of power relations through consumerism and new forms of scientific-bureaucratic knowledge is not the to-be-taken-for-granted outcome that health policies promise. The crucial question is: does the transformation follow the pathway of modernity and the underlying order of a knowledge system based on hierarchy between nature–culture, mind–body, men–women and its many surrogates? Or is this transformation capable of developing a social order of knowledge that contributes to equality, diversity and citizens' participation?

Medical governance and consumerism: introducing new criteria of legitimate knowledge

Consumerism and scientific-bureaucratic medicine not only impact on levels of state regulation and the organisation of health care. They also introduce new criteria of legitimate knowledge and incite competition between different knowledge systems. Bringing users into the equation contributes to the extension of knowledge and confronts biomedical knowledge with new perspectives of lay knowledge. In addition, managerial regulation and performance indicators need new strategies to legitimise knowledge. The title and qualification of a physician, which, in former times, gave access to market power and state protection, no longer guarantee these privileges.

Against the backdrop of marketisation in health care there is an increasing need for reliable data to allow for informed decisions and to improve the safety of patients and the public at large. The explored changes in the building of trust confirm that nowadays the effectiveness and efficiency of the formalised expert system have to be justified using tools borrowed from management, and the 'embodied' knowledge of doctors needs the proof of scientific-bureaucratic medicine (Chapter Eight, this volume). Whether and how the different knowledge systems converge, clash or intersect, and what shifts in power relations are emerging are assessed in the following sections.

Consumerism and the power of medical knowledge

Users, as formerly excluded groups, are increasingly viewed as actors in health care. As citizens they are to be included in regulation and decision-making processes; as patients they are to be treated as fully informed partners of doctors and capable of self-determined decision making. These new actors call for new forms of control of and access to knowledge. For example, Oakley argues that "formalized approaches to knowledge are needed in order to protect the public from the damaging effects of professional and other forms of arrogance" (2000, p 323). A common feature of this debate is that it is more concerned with technological procedures than with the content of knowledge and the expert system on which the body of information is based.

This 'technological' approach to user participation based on improved information and bureaucratic regulation is embedded in health policies and actively taken up by physicians. My data show that physicians are willing to expand patient information and to give proof of quality of their services without, however, including patients' subjectivity and diverse knowledge on health care (Chapters Five and Six, this volume). The medical profession successfully manages to translate new demands for social inclusion and control into a new technology of producing, managing and communicating knowledge.

Paradoxically, one important social effect of consumerism is the strengthening rather than weakening of expert knowledge, and the expansion of professionalism into new fields. While the communication of knowledge formerly took place primarily in the patient–physician interactions, and the 'production' of this knowledge was more or less limited to clinical experiences and biomedical scientific measurements, we now face a much wider range of 'communicators', 'managers' and 'producers' of knowledge. The range includes, for example, consultants from different professions, managers, IT technicians and the media. Furthermore, in the wake of medical governance the production of knowledge is extended to new logic and new arenas, where the legitimacy of knowledge is negotiated between different actors. The innovative aspect is that the creation of knowledge has clearly become more diverse and must therefore be renegotiated.

In all Western societies a paternalistic discourse that allows doctors to decide what it is best for patients to know is being replaced by the discourse of shared decision making that requires fully informed patients (NHS CRD, 1999; Scheibler et al, 2003). My empirical data confirm that physicians and patients take up and transform this discourse; transformations take place on both sides but with different options, aims and interests (Chapters Five and Seven, this volume). If we go beyond discourse and look at practice, however, the limited options of users in the processes of knowledge production become apparent. The findings of this study point to weaknesses and deficits on the levels of health policy and professional practice, but also to limitations that go beyond the scope of mere changes in policies and professional practice. Firstly, neither the decision makers concerned with the macro-level of health policy nor the doctors communicating with patients accept service users as equal players in health care. Secondly, service users are forced to rely, for the main part, on knowledge and information produced by medical professionals within a scope of biomedical research. And, thirdly, biomedical knowledge pervades subjective perceptions.

It is important to note that studies carried out in different health systems and different areas of health care point to similar deficiencies and obstacles. For example, a review of the international literature on shared decision making reveals that "the level of patient preference to participate in decisions is higher than their actual involvement" (Scheibler et al, 2003, p 11). Even in primary care – the core of patient-centred care – the patient's perspective is not well integrated (Sullivan, 2003). Drawing on data from Britain, Newman and Vidler (2006: forthcoming) highlight the fact that patients' needs and wishes are contested concepts, which represents a field of conflict between physicians and patients. This is what the patients in my study described as "then the doctor lets down the shutter [...] because they are not sure of the matter", or "then you don't fit into the system and then it's better if you leave and don't show yourself there anymore" (Chapter Seven, this volume).

Although user involvement in the health policy process has made fair progress in Britain and been significantly improved by "changes in the political environment" (Baggott et al, 2005, p 291), inequalities in the expert–lay divide have not yet been overcome. We can thus conclude that some of the problems are embedded in the consumerist model of regulation itself and cannot be solved satisfactorily by improving the tools and techniques of regulation (Gabe and Calnan, 2000; Clarke et al, 2005).

This assumption is confirmed with respect to a key element of consumerism, namely, the provision of information. My findings reveal that physicians expand patient information but this does not cover the entire spectrum of demands and wishes of patients (Chapters Five and Seven, this volume). A study of information provision in different settings of health care – comprising patient–provider encounters, health promotion programmes and national health policy making, and case studies carried out in the US, Canada, England and Australia – illustrates that deficits in physicians' practice are an outcome of a knowledge system based on dualism (Lee and Garvin, 2003). The authors identify the traditional practice of information transfer in a one-way monologue – in contrast to an exchange of information in a dialogue – as a major problem. Following their interpretation, this practice is related to issues of power, control and the knowledge system: "The association of medicine with natural science and Kantian dualism has allowed for the reifying of scientific knowledge and objectification of the body"

(2003, p 462). It leads to the marginalisation and rejection of lay perspectives.

However, there is – and always has been – resistance to the dominant discourses of biomedical information. The women's health movement and its resistance and challenges to biomedicine is one of the most important instances of this (BWHBC, 1971; see Kuhlmann and Kolip, 2005); the claims of disabled people on the definitions of health and the extension of self-help groups provide further examples. Without doubt, users always voiced their own ideas (Chapter Seven, this volume), but at the same time, the medical profession includes and converts these ideas into a biomedical framework of health care, thereby transforming the knowledge base. Grassroot movements enhance significant changes in health care systems and medical practice, and promote diversity of knowledge, but they do not substantively weaken medical power. It is important to understand the high flexibility of professionalism and the fluidity of boundaries between different players and knowledge systems in order to assess the impact of new regulatory policies and changing user demands (for instance, for alternative therapies and new communication styles between doctors and patients).

Struggles over legitimate knowledge not only occur in the expert–lay relationship, they are also vivid in the decision making of individual patients. I described this as the 'seeping' of biomedical knowledge into individual perceptions (Chapter Seven, this volume). Biomedical knowledge 'colonialised' Western culture from the beginning of the professionalisation of medicine in the 18th century and began to pervade individual perceptions. Although the women's health movement and the biomedical counterculture of the 1960s and 1970s brought the suppression of self-knowledge and alternative knowledge systems and its negative impact on health and well-being into view, 'colonialisation' is still at work. It is even reinforced in some areas of health care, like medical genetics (Kuhlmann, 2002).

The freedom to choose information from a variety of sources and knowledge systems does not easily change the cultural consensus on the supremacy of biomedicine. For example, patients in my focus groups most valued information given by a physician (Chapter Seven, this volume). Under these conditions, the 'choice' and 'self-determination' of patients and the public are shaped by a powerful biomedical discourse and its embeddedness in the institutions of health care. The concept of choice therefore needs to be set in the context of cultural and institutional environments.

Further limitations of a consumerist model of participation become apparent when we look at the ambiguous and even contradictory demands and wishes of patients. As described in Chapter Seven, the patients in my study claimed 'self-determined' decisions in some situations while they wished for a doctor's advice and help in others. They redefine the concept of choice in ways that cross the divide between 'autonomy' and 'dependency'. Similarly, in a study of doctor—patient relations in Australia some years ago, Lupton (1997) concluded that although patients adopt consumerist behaviour in some contexts, in others they prefer to take doctors' advice. The author detects a subtle pressure being brought to bear on patients to adopt a consumerist position and to suppress "their equally strongly felt desire at other times to take on a 'passive patient' role and invest their trust and faith in these professionals" (1997, p 380).

Improved user involvement on macro and micro-levels of decision making does not therefore cover the entire range of demands on social inclusion and participation. Sullivan argues for an incorporation of patients' subjectivity into medical evaluations that "should carry us well beyond informed consent and the other protections for patient autonomy" (2003, p 1595). He criticises the 'value-free' perspective of clinical medicine that is "rooted in natural science, even though caring for patients requires many other forms of knowledge" (2003, p 1602). Accordingly, the problems go far beyond the regulation and practice of the medical profession and touch on the epistemological foundations of Western culture.

Sustainable changes cannot be expected to simply emerge from the expansion and pluralisation of information nor from structural changes related to improved user participation. There is a need to redefine medical theories of the body, illness and disease (Bendelow et al, 2002; Williams, 2003), and to critically review the claims on neutrality and objectivity of medical knowledge. The subject—object and lay—expert divide is open to discussion. This calls for new methods and measurements of quality and efficiency that move beyond the mere 'trust in numbers' (Porter, 1995) towards a redefinition of objectivity that takes account of the diversity of citizens' needs and wishes.

Standardisation of knowledge and the production of objectivity

Standardisation of knowledge is an important tool of new governance in health care. Performance indicators are well on the way to becoming an essential instrument of political control (Schepers and Casparie, 1999; Exworthy et al, 2003), and EBM represents the 'gold standard' against which all decision making in health care is measured (Timmermans and Berg, 2003). Taking over my argument outlined in the previous chapter, regulatory power is not derived solely from the broad acceptance of the tools themselves, but from the shared belief in the information and the underlying knowledge system.

New regulatory patterns rely on the power of seemingly objective and neutralised information and "well-designed empirical ways of knowing" (Oakley, 2000, p 312) to transform the relationship between professions and service users. This approach ignores the fact that it is the members of the medical profession who develop these designs, carry out the research and produce the evidence on which policy decisions are based. The standardisation of care through clinical guidelines and EBM provides new opportunities for the medical profession to apply the technique they know best; and physicians' voices are the strongest when it comes to deciding what is 'evident' and what is not, even under managerial conditions (Timmermans and Berg, 2003). Blank and Burau (2004, p 137) call this "the rebirth of medical practice" in the wake of quality management, and emphasise that we should not simply expect a revival but new dimensions of this practice.

The promises of provider control and user participation that are embedded in new models of governing health care cannot necessarily be supported by empirical data (Chapters Six and Seven, this volume). The space for making legitimate knowledge and transforming it into power relations in health care may be more expanded under conditions of corporatist regulation in Germany than by state-centred and market-driven regulation. There are, however, striking similarities in the empirical studies from different health systems in that they all point to significant limitations of new patterns aimed at managing and controlling professional knowledge.

Medical governance provokes much controversy over 'cookbook medicine' and such like, and without doubt, enhances frontline changes in health care. However, the medical profession continues to govern the production, management and communication of knowledge. McDonald and Harrison conclude from developments in the NHS that participation in the guideline process "functioned primarily as a device by which actors hoped to pursue their existing opinion, either through imposing them on others, or by creating a framework of legitimation for themselves" (2004, p 223). The new elements of medical governance, therefore, remain weak drivers for sustainable change in health care systems (Chapter Four, this volume).

The potential of EBM to strengthen medical power, instead of weakening it, lies in the knowledge base and the claims for authority of science and unique truth. Harrison critically highlights the underlying questionable assumptions of EBM:

> The model is deterministic (that is, it assumes that clinical events necessarily have causes which can be identified and, in principle, modified) and realist or naturalist (that is, it entails a belief in a world of objectively real entities whose nature can be observed). (1998, pp 25-6)

Harrison puts EBM in the context of social change and regulation, and outlines the ties with Fordism. As "a late flower of Fordism" it is related to the ideology of rationalism and a single 'best way' of production, and seems to run "against the tide of the times" (1998, p 26).

This perspective draws attention to the ties – rather than the contradictions – between scientific biomedical knowledge and managerial and economic knowledge. Both knowledge systems are based on paradigms of neutrality and objectivity. Both are reductionist and positivist in claiming the one and only truth, thereby excluding diversity, subjectivity and the context of knowledge production and use. The merger of medical science and managerial tools to scientific-bureaucratic medicine are a perfect tool with which to eliminate subjectivity and context, and even intensify the 'conquering gaze' (Haraway, 1991) of biomedicine. For example, claims of evidence-based data and orthodox research methods are often used to legitimise the exclusion of CAM therapies (Kelner et al, 2004) and the marginalisation of gender issues and women's health care needs (Eckman, 1998).

Strengthening EBM in health policy and practice is celebrated as a victory of formalisation and cognitive criteria over the limited knowledge base of individual clinical experience and the qualification of physicians. The 'production of objectivity' and the 'rationalisation' of knowledge are key issues in EBM. Science and practice are thus placed in a hierarchical order that devalues the embodied knowledge – of patients as well as providers – and the clinical experience of physicians. This interpretation appears to be yet another variation of the age-old debate on the supremacy of mind over body, and suchlike (Knorr-Cetina, 1981; Latour and Woolgar, 1986; Haraway, 1991), which are used to underpin exclusion and hierarchy. However, the new tools to standardise care and manage the knowledge production in health care are part of reflexive processes of modernisation: they carry the problems of modernity and Western knowledge, and at the same time provide new opportunities to transform the knowledge system and improve social participation.

Transforming the knowledge system

Following the official definition of EBM given by Sackett and his co-authors (1997), this practice is described as integrating individual clinical experience with the best available external clinical evidence, which is conducted from RCTs, meta-analysis and systematic reviews of the medical literature. According to this definition, EBM is not simply the imposition of clinical and subjective experience but its systematic accumulation in order to achieve higher quality and safety. Viewed through this lens it should be clear that EBM incorporates the entire underlying cognitive framework and 'binary thinking' of medicine. Although it comes out on top as the new paradigm and downplays its tensions with discretionary, context-based clinical decision making, it does not overcome medical and bioethical uncertainty (Fox, 2002).

Greer (1998) outlines the fundamentally different goals and cultures of science and practice, and insists that while complexity might be reduced to the level of scientific guidelines, it cannot be eliminated from clinical practice. The care of individual patients always calls for context-sensitive decisions. EBM has clearly incorporated the structural ambivalence of science and clinical practice through its reliance on clinical data (Harrison, 1998). There is a clear and urgent need for transparency in decision making and for a reduction of unintended variety, but there is no need for a 'one-size-fits-all' standard and unique truth of biomedical evidence (Best and Glik, 2003). Moreover, there is a need for a re-evaluation of qualitative research and a context-based framework that takes the utilisation of evidence into consideration (Grol et al, 2002; Dean, 2004; Dobrow et al, 2004).

In part, the introduction of scientific-bureaucratic medicine runs counter to knowledge diversity – even within the medical profession – and the participation of patients and citizens in decision making. The cognitive basis and the methodological tools are related to a traditional knowledge paradigm that tends to exclude all those who do not fit the dominant standard. The patients in my study were well aware of these problems when they expressed their fears that their individual situation does not "fit the standards", and that they would not, therefore, receive the care they needed (Chapter Seven, this volume). EBM, as the key of scientific-bureaucratic medicine, is a powerful tool to 'produce' knowledge and put it into a legitimised system of formalised procedures. This tool is reinforced by managerial procedures but remains, for most of the time, in the hands of the medical profession (Chapters Five and Six, this volume).

At the same time, increasing formalisation and the need to legitimise medical knowledge and decision making make the pitfalls and shortcomings of biomedicine apparent. In doing so it nurtures critical approaches from within and from outside the medical profession. Critique with regard to gender bias in highly formalised procedures of knowledge production (Healy, 1991), such as RCTs and evidence-based clinical guidelines, and recent changes in these procedures, provide striking examples of the opportunities of new regulatory tools to remake medical knowledge and create a more gender-sensitive knowledge base (Kuhlmann and Kolip, 2005). These and other transformations provoke fissures in the knowledge system, which, in turn, generate and nurture new patterns of professionalism. These processes open pathways for new 'knowers' and the chance to introduce new and to re-evaluate existing criteria of legitimate knowledge – however tentative the character of these changes may be at present. The crucial point is whether the enhanced dynamics actually lead to a loosening of the knowledge–power knot as the key of the power of the medical profession and how these dynamics could be fostered.

Unravelling the knowledge–power knot of professionalism

Empirical findings indicate that the two key elements of new regulatory models, consumerism and managerialism in their various forms, do not cover the entire range of the knowledge–power knot and the options to loosen it. An important limitation of new governance is that it introduces managerial criteria but does not radically transform the knowledge system. A changing dramaturgy of governance in health care does not, therefore, tell us whether professions play their new role less successfully than hitherto. The ambivalence incorporated in the concepts of consumerism and evidence-based policy and practice opens up various ways for the medical profession to make use of new claims on legitimate knowledge without radically changing the balance of power. The physicians in my study were well aware of the new options. Despite their sometimes ambiguous feelings towards standards and guidelines, physicians make use of these tools to give public proof of the quality of their services; they also significantly improved patient information (Chapter Six, this volume).

Fissures in the knowledge–power knot of professionalism may widen if changes in different dimensions of knowledge–power relations point in the same direction. At present, dynamics are especially enhanced by the improved participation of users and a growing interest in CAM therapies. Both areas of change significantly challenge the supremacy of biomedical knowledge. Strong dynamics can be expected if improved user participation, claims for other than biomedical treatment and the professionalisation of providers of these therapies amalgamate. In this case, the biomedical knowledge system and the power of its representatives would be challenged on different levels: it would have to react to the self-knowledge of patients and new demands on providers, on the one hand, and the various knowledge claims of CAM therapists, on the other.

Accordingly, the advancement of new professional projects and shifts in the system of professions may be a source and strategy to change knowledge–power relations and improve the accountability of professions in the interests of citizens. Midwifery provides convincing examples of the success of such a strategy (Bourgeault et al, 2004; Chapter One, this volume). Professionalisation may thus serve as a potential for innovation rather than a conservative force and barrier to change.

However, new players and regulatory tools do not necessarily shift the power away from the medical profession. The biomedical expert knowledge system does not merely derive power from its formalisation but from multiple and intertwined levels – structure, action and culture. The impact of new governance thus depends on context. In this respect, institutional environments model the conditions of change – as the differences, for instance in gender-sensitive performance indicators in the US and the German health system indicate (Chapter Two, this volume). Accordingly, the state is an important actor when it comes to the resources that enable diverse – and, with respect to social, economic and cultural resources, different – actors in health care to participate as equal players in the negotiation on knowledge claims. Despite the many efforts to improve the control of providers, the alliance between the government and the medical profession remains strong in all Western countries when it comes to biomedical knowledge, as this provides the most powerful and most trusted source to legitimate policies and decision making in health care.

A further condition of change in the knowledge–power knot of professionalism is change in the cultural consensus of the supremacy of biomedical knowledge. This can be enhanced through congruence between public interests and interest-based strategies of new occupational groups striving for professionalisation. Here again, the wished-for alliance between the government and the service user on the one hand, and conflict of interests between professionals and users on the other, is only one of the possible outcomes. Claims for the inclusion of CAM therapies in Statutory Health in Germany, as well as claims for safe information apart from that given by physicians, provide examples of conflicting interests of the users and those of the government to contain costs (Chapter Seven, this volume). In this situation the alliance of the government and the medical profession is a more likely outcome than the improvement of user choice and diversity of health care services.

The findings make the shortcomings of neoliberal logic that underpins new governance apparent: they challenge the assumptions on conflicting interests between the professions and the state, and between providers and users. In all likelihood, the interests of the various players are related in more complex ways, and the outcome of new regulatory models is not always necessarily in line with health policy incentives. An example of the messy and uneven processes of change is provided in the potentially adverse effects of the building of trust in institutions without damaging trust in doctors (Chapter Eight, this volume). The capacity of the medical profession to 'conquer' an innovative potential of new governance in order to bypass tighter public control gives further proof that professionalism is malleable according to new demands (Chapters Five and Six, this volume).

This leads us back to the interface between professions, the state and the public, and the key role of the professions as mediators. The power of biomedical knowledge is not unconditional. It is stabilised by a pattern of state regulation that privileges biomedical knowledge in the health system and the position of the medical profession in the stakeholder arrangement; and it is also stabilised by citizens' trust in doctors and a cultural consensus on the supremacy of medical knowledge. Governments of all Western countries increasingly include users in the health policy process but allow for an ongoing biomedical 'colonialisation' of the health systems. This is perhaps the most powerful conservative force in health care across the Western world.

A new pattern of governing the medical profession by using managerial tools is only one of the possible options to loosen the knowledge–power knot. Bringing new actors and diversity of interests into the equation of regulatory arrangements may provoke deeper fissures and more sustainable shifts in the knowledge system and the balance of power in health care. These strategies are stronger drivers for change, and here we can observe considerable differences between the health systems (Chapter Four, this volume). Such a 'modernised' pattern of governance based on coordination and negotiation of diverse interests and demands of the service users and the entire health workforce could target the transformations of professions towards better accountability to the interests of various members of the public.

TEN

Conclusion

This book set out to assess the dynamics of the modernisation processes in health care. The study highlighted the interconnectedness and tensions between the professions, the state and the public, which release ongoing dynamics and new uncertainty into the policy process and practice of health care. We cannot understand change in health care without looking at professions as mediators between the state and its citizens, and empirically studying their options and strategies to shape the reform processes under way in all health systems. At the same time, the regulatory framework of the state and the role of service users are crucial to better understanding the advancement of professionals more accountable to the public. However, welfare state categories of market, state or corporatist regulation are no longer sustainable. More hybrid modes of governing health care call for new theoretical approaches that move beyond institutional regulation, and for empirical data. The contribution of this study is to assess the global phenomena of modernisation in a new context of conservative corporatist regulation; it hereby allows for a critical review of the currently dominant reform models and turns the spotlight onto new policy options. It also brings into view a broader range of drivers and enablers of modernisation processes in health care. In summarising the findings I will focus on three issues: the rise of a new professionalism; the released tensions and dynamics in the triangle of the professions, the state and the public; and the potential of corporatism and professional self-regulation for modernisation.

Varieties of professionalism in late modernity

Developments within the medical profession and the health occupations clearly indicate that professionalism is becoming more diverse and context-dependent. New patterns of professionalism, new strategies to promote professional interest, and new patterns of professional identity are observed in the medical profession as the archetype of a profession, and also in occupational groups that strive for professionalisation, such as physiotherapists.

The emergence of managerialism and networks and more

contextualised identities indicates that changes are under way in the structure, action and culture of the medical profession (Chapters Five and Six, this volume). Physicians feel a need to overcome "encrusted" patterns of SHI regulation and "stiff grandfathers" and "bureaucrats", as some participants in my study expressed it. They are calling for the modernisation of medical self-regulation from the bottom up, but they do not aim to replace corporatist institutions. The medical profession – commonly viewed as a conservative actor – takes up and transforms elements from new governance aimed at controlling providers into successful strategies to promote its own professional interests. The key areas where changes are manifest include quality management, coordination of provider services and patient information. The improvement of coordination through networks and more participatory bottom-up structures of decision making release dynamics into the governance process, the organisation of health care and the health workforce, that may contribute to modernisation processes and social inclusion). Consequently, professions do not necessarily act as conservative forces; they also enable change.

The rise of new patterns of professionalism is equally striking with regard to the health occupations. Classic strategies aimed at advancing the transformation of an occupational group into a profession are not available for these groups in Germany, especially state protection and market closure. Moreover, the health occupations apply hybrid strategies based on various elements of professionalism and individualised tactics of market power. However, the examples of physiotherapists – and surgery receptionists in particular – underscore the limitations of such tactics. On top of this, there is a lack of collective strategies aimed at inclusion in the legal framework of SHI regulation.

This weakness mirrors the problems of gendered tactics of professionalisation that focus on change in the workplace and 'credentialism' rather than legalistic tactics. Consequently, both groups cannot effectively make use of the new opportunities provided by a policy discourse of integrated care and cooperation. Health reform in Germany turns out to be neither a facilitator in the professionalisation of physiotherapy nor a 'job machine' for surgery receptionists, although it does provide new opportunities for individuals to improve market power. Even though the use of a discourse of professionalism is spreading to new occupational groups, this does not necessarily mean that it can be applied successfully.

There is evidence for a rise of a new professionalism in the wake of new governance and changing concepts of citizenship, which is significantly different from earlier forms (Larson, 1977). New forms of professionalism advance cooperation, render boundaries within and between occupational groups more permeable, and enable more contextualised identities. Interestingly, transformations of citizenship and claims for participation do not simply act as external forces, like user participation; they can be also observed within the medical profession. At the same time, there is evidence for the persistence of classic patterns of professionalism based on exclusion, demarcation and hierarchy. For example, negative attitudes of physicians regarding cooperation with the health occupations or patient rights are proof of the legacy of exclusionary tactics and hegemonic claims (Chapter Five, this volume). Empirical findings reveal that classic strategies of exclusion and new patterns of a more inclusive professionalism are applied simultaneously (Table 10.1).

Table 10.1: Diversity of professionalism between exclusion and social inclusion

Exclusionary patterns of professionalism	→ ←	More inclusive patterns of professionalism
Hierarchical, bureaucratic patterns of self-regulation and self-administration	→ ←	Network governance, more active participation in the self-regulatory bodies
Striving for market closure	→ ←	Cooperation
'Tribalism' and occupational closure	→ ←	Networking and more permeable occupational boundaries
Claims for 'autonomy' and self-determined decision making	→ ←	Inclusion of managerialism, standardisation of care, EBM
Quality of care based on individual qualification	→ ←	Quality of care based on formalised procedures and performance indicators
Identity construction based on 'belonging' to a professional community	→ ←	More contextualised and permeable identity constructions
Gendered division of the health workforce	→ ←	Changing gender relations within professions
Expert–lay divide	→ ←	Improved information, inclusion of users in regulatory bodies
Professionalism restricted to the medical and other high-status occupational groups	→ ←	Health occupations refer to professionalism to upgrade occupational status

Exclusionary and more inclusive patterns of professionalism do not simply co-exist. They release new dynamics that lead to a greater diversity of professionalism. Existing overlaps and tensions between conflicting patterns of professionalism enhance various new forms of promoting professional interests. However, greater diversity plays out differently in different occupational groups, as has been shown for the three groups studied here (Chapter Six, this volume). Although each group is renegotiating its place in the health system, the medical profession has the greatest ability to flexibly combine classic and new patterns of professionalism, and to develop new strategies to successfully promote professional interests. Awareness of the varieties and tensions between conservative and innovative elements of professionalism is crucial to arrive at a better understanding of the options and barriers inherent in the new models of governing health care, and the medical profession's room for manoeuvre.

New governance in health care: tensions and instabilities in the triangle of the professions, the state and the public

The state increasingly takes on a more active role in the regulation of health care. New policy approaches apply elements of new governance and more clearly intervene in the organisation of care. The twin strategies of managerialism – or more specifically, medical governance (Gray and Harrison, 2004) – and improved user participation are expected to reduce the power of providers, particularly medicine, and to improve public control. However, the findings of this study indicate that the effects are more complex and may play out in ways not intended by health policies.

Characteristic of new governance approaches is an ongoing hybridisation between professional self-regulation and managerial control. Contrary to common expectations, however, the medical profession itself is an important force that advances more hybrid forms of regulation. Physicians increasingly amalgamate managerialism and professionalism (Chapters Five and Six, this volume). They make use of managerial tools – such as EBM, clinical guidelines and quality assurance – as new 'signifiers' of quality of care and a new 'technology' of building trust in medical services (Chapter Eight, this volume). They are thus capable of ensuring public trust in doctors under changing conditions and, most importantly, outflanking tighter public control and the establishment of a comprehensive system of accountability. A global discourse of citizenship and user participation is translated into an individual discourse of 'patient-centred care' and 'patient information'; in other words, it remains under the control of the medical profession.

Similar effects can be observed at the level of organisation of providers. A policy goal of merging providers into networks is translated into a new strategy of promoting physicians' interests through networking and cooperation (Chapter Six, this volume). These developments underscore the flexibility and transformability of professionalism: the boundaries between market logic, bureaucracy and professionalism – the 'third logic', as Freidson (2001) calls it – are permeable and fluid rather than solid and static.

The options for transformations are especially strong in Germany as no established system of accountability and managerial control exists; there are no powerful actors who could exercise this control effectively. In contrast to the NHS managers in the British system and the MCO in the US, the options of the SHI funds in Germany are more limited in terms of the statutory framework of corporatist regulation. In particular, SHI funds cannot directly intervene in the organisation of care. New models have to be negotiated in the public law institutions, which means that agreement must be sought with physicians. The moderate changes in the organisation of care observed in my study confirm that the dynamics of new governance may impact within the medical profession (Chapter Five, this volume). But they do not significantly change the system of health professions and occupations or the core of corporatist regulation, namely, the centrality of the physicians' associations and SHI funds. However, we cannot predict accurately whether, and how, policy makers, SHI funds or the health occupations will use managerial tools more effectively in future, and what the role of users will be. But we should be prepared for unintended dynamics that may even run contradictory to the policy aims.

Results of my study lead to the conclusion that the German government cannot rely on patients as partners to control health care providers. Efforts to introduce new models of care tend to be viewed with suspicion, and are overshadowed by patient concerns. It is not likely that the users will support the policy attempts of strengthening the role of SHI funds against physicians' associations. Moreover, the SHI funds are perceived as economic organisations rather than 'advocates' of patient interests (Chapter Seven, this volume). That means that a keystone of the Bismarckian system, namely, the delegation of user interests to the SHI funds as counterparts of the medical profession, is no longer sustainable.

Although user power is weak on the institutional level, the interplay of dynamics on different levels and in different areas of health care may provoke unintended changes. As a consequence, consumerism may prove to be a greater challenge to the state than to the professions. Users place new demands on the government to provide the resources for them to exercise their new role as 'expert patients' and 'discriminating consumers' (Newman and Vidler, 2006: forthcoming). Examples of this are the calls for information centres independent from physicians and SHI funds, comprehensive information on treatment options not limited to biomedicine, and safety of the information. In contrast to development in the NHS (Baggott et al, 2005; Davies et al, 2005), for instance, the German government does not adequately respond to these demands. Consumerism provides another example that a global discourse on reform is transformed in nation-specific ways and may thus play out differently.

Furthermore, providers and service users may form new alliances not intended by health policy, especially when it comes to the 'freedom of choice' of a provider and treatment options. 'Choice' is structurally embedded in the classic model of SHI care and a highly held cultural value in society at large. Combined with high levels of trust in doctors and the power of biomedical knowledge, such alliances may even strengthen the powerful position of the medical profession. Germany's physician-centred reform models – like the DMPs and the gatekeeper models of office-based generalists – may encourage rather than deter such alliances.

However, such alliances cannot simply be viewed as a conservative force that strengthens medical power; they may also generate pressure for alternative agendas to be raised. We know from the success of the women's health movement that users are capable of voicing their demands and building alliances in ways that can lead to structural changes in health care systems. The increasing calls of patients for CAM and for better and safer information may release similar dynamics in the future, which could result in complex changes in the workforce and SHI care. As described at length elsewhere, a comparative study of Britain and Germany (Newman and Kuhlmann, 2007: forthcoming) reveals that consumers may act in ways that were not intended and that might be beyond governments' control.

In the Introduction I set out a research model that places the professions as mediators between the state and citizens. Research now reveals that new policy aims of creating 'citizen professionals' more accountable to the public do not simply impact on the professions in a linear sequence. Moreover, they change the mediating role of professions in complex and even unintended ways. This enhances new

Figure 10.1: Professions, the state and the public as a dynamic triangle

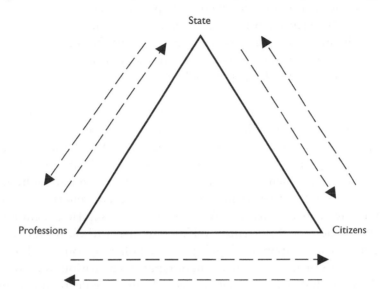

tensions in the triangle comprising professions, the state and the public, and consequently, the relationships are becoming more dynamic (Figure 10.1). In particular, 'citizen consumers' put new demands on the government, and 'citizen professionals' create new models of coordination and self-regulation. New governance not only challenges medical power and changes professionalism; it also challenges and changes the concepts of both state and public. In doing so, it creates new instabilities in the governance of health care.

Renewal of corporatism: moving beyond medical governance

The first two sections to this chapter looked to the professions as mediators and thereby directed attention to the dynamics in the wider health system and the role of the state. This section further outlines the importance of regulatory frameworks and the challenges of health reform models. Different health systems of market-driven, state-centred or corporatist regulation increasingly show overlaps in the modes of governing health care:

> The European and American models are becoming a bit more like the British one. In France, for example, social insurance contributions are now buttressed by a general

tax on income. In America, a big expansion of government spending on older people to help pay for their drugs bills will be financed from general tax revenues. And in Britain, Mr Brown pushed up social insurance contributions in his 2002 budget to raise money for the surge in spending on the NHS. (*The Economist*, 18 August 2005)

The findings of my study confirm an ongoing hybridisation of regulatory models, but they also reveal that different models do not simply converge. Viewing the reform processes in health care through a country-specific and less Anglo–American lens brings into view more sustainable changes in the professions and new options for health policy. It is interesting to note here that a recent report from the Anglo–German Foundation (AGF, 2005) draws similar conclusions on the capacity of the German welfare system as a whole for renewal. A contextualised approach highlights new policy options to advance modernisation in a way that encourages participation and social inclusion of hitherto marginal players in health care decision making and practice. I argued that major obstacles of modernisation not only derive from professional politics and the hegemonic claims of the medical profession. Moreover, conservative forces are also embedded in the corporatist system and shaped by state regulation ('path dependency'; see Chapters Three and Four, this volume).

Both health occupations studied here indicate that limited options – to professionalise in the case of physiotherapists or to improve self-determined work and occupational chances in the case of surgery receptionists – are not simply a matter of medical dominance. Over and above this, limitations are an outcome of a lack of state support and exclusion from the main regulatory bodies. In this respect the findings from health occupations in Germany echo Saks' (2003b) conclusion from research into CAM practitioners in Britain and the US, namely, that comprehensive regulatory frameworks may promote the inclusion of new approaches and actors in health care (Chapter One, this volume). Accordingly, a more plural legal framework and policy approach can be identified as a strong driver of modernisation processes, but one that is marginal in the global discourse of reform, and particularly ignored in Germany. In contrast to cost containment – the dominant policy driver across countries – this driver advances more 'enabling' processes of change. It may further social inclusion and participation of all those who are less powerful and labelled 'others' in the arena of biomedicine.

Furthermore, and also related to state regulation, the 'gender of professions' (Davies, 1996) remains a powerful conservative force even in times of a policy discourse of integrated caring concepts and equal opportunity. The predominantly female health occupations have no say when it comes to the negotiation of reform models and the definition of standards and 'evidence' of treatment options. They also lack the qualifications and resources to fulfil the new demands, and they apply gendered strategies to advance a professional project by employing 'credentialist' tactics, which are less successful than legalistic tactics (Witz, 1992). This circle of disadvantages continuously enables the medical profession to fill the gaps and to remake the knowledge–power knot of professionalism.

It is the coming together of conservative forces in different areas of social policy that creates and reinforces conservative elements in the governing of health care: firstly, conservatism in the health system, like the limited stakeholder arrangement of SHI regulation; secondly, in the training system, particularly in the lack of multidisciplinary training concepts and career options for health occupations; and, thirdly, in society at large, like gender hierarchy, traditional gender identities and an institutionalised 'male breadwinner model'. Consequently, the persistence of conservative elements and blockades towards modernisation cannot be changed substantively by tighter regulation of the medical profession. It calls for complex changes to be made in the regulatory system, including both intersectorial and gender-sensitive social policy approaches.

The most crucial outcome of conservatism of the German health system is the lack of acknowledgement of all health care workers and their exclusion from key regulatory bodies. These deficiencies impact like a cascade on the health system and seriously limit the overall scope for reform. The regulatory framework reproduces a physician-centred health system; the transformation of integrated caring concepts and primary care approaches into its German version of cooperation of medical providers, like DMPs, or a gatekeeper system of office-based generalists, are proof of its limitations.

Furthermore, it limits interprofessional dynamics and synergetic forces towards a 'learning system' of cooperation. Such dynamics could be generated, for example, by the greater willingness of some physicians' networks to cooperate with health occupations, or by a more positive attitude towards multidisciplinary care on the part of physiotherapists and feminist providers of health care (Chapter Six, this volume).

We cannot then understand the structural rigidities of the German system by simply looking at medical governance and the effects of the self-regulation of physicians. Instead, the state is also a key actor, or an 'architect' (Döhler, 1995) in terms of the welfare state, when it comes to supporting the professionalisation of the health occupations and integrated caring models based on primary care as defined by the WHO (Chapter Two, this volume). Despite a wide-ranging debate on reform, there is at present no sign that the German government is moving in this direction. Although health policy attempts to weaken medical power, in actual fact it contributes to its continuity. The increasing need to legitimise unpopular decisions, especially the exclusion of services from SHI care and increasingly limited options for patients to choose a provider, may even reinforce unintended alliances. The knowledge–power knot of professionalism might thus be strengthened rather than weakened. In particular, EBM and biomedical knowledge provide the most powerful tools for legitimising policy decisions; they enjoy the highest levels of acceptance among the different social groups that make up the public (Chapter Nine, this volume).

Health reform policies in Germany make use of weak drivers for modernisation, like managerialism, but ignore two strong drivers, namely comprehensive regulation of the health occupations and a primary care approach (Chapter Four, this volume). Despite the government's new willingness to move to the front of the stage, as demonstrated from the health reforms in 2000 and onwards and reinforced by the 2004 Health Modernisation Act, corporatist regulation has not substantively been changed (Chapter Three, this volume). Consequently, room for manoeuvre is greatest in those areas where the position of the medical profession is at its strongest: the negotiations on the organisation of providers and quality management.

There are clear signs that the German government is attempting to limit the medical profession's scope of action. However, these attempts bear the mark of classic corporatist regulation and physician-centred reform models. Change is expected primarily from shifting the balance of power within the medical profession towards generalists, and within the regulatory system towards SHI funds. Although service users are now included in the regulatory system, the focus remains on physicians and SHI funds. The government fails to support the establishment of a structure of bottom-up decision making of user representatives, and the inclusion of users in all stages and areas of the policy process (Chapter Seven, this volume). In particular, the newly established Institute of Quality and Efficiency in Health Care gives proof of a strategy that aims at enabling neither 'voice' nor agency of the service users, nor of the health occupations. Moreover, it nurtures a strategy of patient-centred care and patient information governed by the medical profession. A lack of more plural policies and regulatory bodies that include the entire spectrum of health care workers and improve participation of service users enables the medical profession to fill the vacancies and maintain power under changing conditions.

However, the recent extension of the Federal Committee and inclusion of user representatives are slowly permeating the monolith of physicians' associations and SHI funds, and opening the door to further changes. The core idea of corporatist regulation, and the SHI system in particular, namely that of governing through a network of public law institutions (Moran, 1999), provides the opportunity to transform a highly efficient model of the 20th century – in terms of compulsory health care, social equality and stability – into a more hybrid network structure of coordination of the diverse players. The crucial issue is that the government does not use these options consistently.

In Chapter Four I explored strong and weak drivers for modernisation from a comparative perspective and traced their application to the German health system. Research shows that the renewal of corporatism provides greater opportunities for modernisation than are currently being taken up in the scope of health policy. Changing patterns of medical governance are only one of the possible options to bring about the policy aims of accountability of professionals, quality of care and user participation. Moreover, more plural regulatory bodies may advance social inclusion of the various health care workers and the service users. They may also act as a 'buffer' against conflicts of interest and new instabilities in state regulation.

The advancement of professionals more accountable to the public calls for the advancement of professionalisation of the health occupations and their acknowledgement as professions; it also requires more empowering consumer policies. The challenge to the state is to develop a more plural regulatory framework to better coordinate the various nation-specific 'knots' and 'enabling players' of modernisation processes within the professions.

Outlook

This study has highlighted the uneven and contorted dynamics of new governance approaches in a corporatist system. At the same time, research indicates that tensions between professions, the state and the public are embedded in professional projects across different health systems and their models of governing professions and the public sphere. Governments of different welfare states may respond differently to new demands in health care; however, change in one relationship in the triangle inevitably creates dynamics that may impact on others. This means there is a need for new – theoretical and political – approaches that move beyond institutional regulation and direct attentions towards actors, agency and context, and the various ways of making and remaking governance (Clarke, 2004; Burau, 2005; Newman, 2005b). There is also a need to reinvent a 'system of professions' (Abbott, 1988) and to make way for different forms of professionalism and 'different avenues' (Saks, 2003b) so that occupational groups hitherto excluded from the system of professions can choose to professionalise. And there is an equally important need to investigate 'the public interest' (Saks, 1995) or 'people' (Newman, 2005a) in both the study of professions and health policy.

My contribution to understanding the dynamics of changing health care systems is to link approaches from the sociology of professions to social policy and health care research, and empirically assess provider and user perspectives and interprofessional dynamics. I argue the need for contextualised approaches that grasp the reflexivity of change in different dimensions and between different players in health care: global patterns of reform and national pathways of institutional and cultural modes of regulation; changing health policies and interest-based strategies of the various professions; and changing relationships between different occupational groups and between providers and users. Placing health professions in the context of changing modes of governance and citizenship brings into view both an innovative potential embedded in professional projects and the role of the state in targeting the outcome of interest-based strategies of the professions.

Professions are appointed to play the double role of public 'officer' and public 'servant' (Bertilsson, 1990; Chapter One, this volume). Whether and how the balance shifts towards the servant – whom I call 'citizen professional' – is to no small degree a matter of state regulation. At the same time, path dependency does not give us the whole story of how the health professions perform their role as mediators. Moreover, alliances between the professions, the state and an increasingly diverse public may enhance new and unintended dynamics. Accordingly, neither path dependency in terms of welfare states nor a debate on the convergence or submergence of national welfare states can actually grasp the dynamics of the process under way in health care. This is also true for approaches that configure the professions as stable rather than malleable occupational groups. Moreover, there is a need for empirical research and questions such as these: how do professions respond to and shape changing welfare state governance? And in turn, how do states govern the professionalisation, politics and practice of professional groups, and how do they empower the 'voice' of service users? And in what ways does this contribute to a 21st-century society's needs and demands on citizenship, social inclusion and diversity? In what way does it improve the quality of health care and public safety?

Set against the backdrop of a strongly self-regulating medical profession and the backstage position adopted by the state, options to either promote or block the modernisation of health care may be especially strong for the medical profession, and the agency of the health occupations especially weak in Germany. However, particular elements of professional self-regulation and corporatism, together with the centrality of medical governance, are important components of all health systems, however state-centred or market-driven they may be. Expanding the scope of research and theories hitherto dominated by Anglo-American approaches contributes to a better understanding of the context dependency of medical power and the significance of regulatory frameworks. Most importantly, a greater diversity of professional projects of formerly subordinated health care workers and more plural regulatory bodies may counteract the hegemonic claims of the medical profession in more sustainable ways than marketisation and managerialism. This approach brings into view a new policy option in the scenario of 'reform' in health care, but one that challenges health politics and policy in complex ways.

References

Abbott, A. (1988) *The system of professions*, Chicago, IL, and London: Chicago University Press.

Abbott, A. (2001) 'What do cases do?', in A. Abbott (ed) *Time matters: On theory and method*, Chicago, IL: University of Chicago Press, pp 129-60.

Abraham, J. (1997) 'The science and politics of medicines' regulation', in M.A. Elston (ed) *The sociology of medical science and technology*, London: Blackwell, pp 153-82.

AGF (Anglo-German Foundation) (2005) 'Publications' (www.agf.org.uk/pubs/publications.shtml).

Ahern, M.M. and Hendryx, M.S. (2003) 'Social capital and trust in providers', *Social Science and Medicine*, vol 57, pp 1195-203.

Alber, J. (1992) *Das Gesundheitswesen der Bundesrepublik Deutschland*, Frankfurt: CAMpus.

Allsop, J. (1999) 'Identity maintenance under conditions of change: the medical profession in the UK in the late twentieth century', in I. Hellberg, M. Saks and C. Benoit (eds) *Professional identities in transition: Cross-cultural dimensions*, Goteborg: Almquist & Wiksell International, pp 157-73.

Allsop, J. and Jones, K. (2006: forthcoming) 'The regulation of health care professions: towards greater partnership between the state, professions and citizens in the UK', *Knowledge, Work & Society*, vol 4, no 1.

Allsop, J. and Saks, M. (eds) (2002a) *Regulating the health professions*, London: Sage Publications.

Allsop, J. and Saks, M. (2002b) 'Introduction', in J. Allsop and M. Saks (eds) *Regulating the health professions*, London: Sage Publications, pp 1-16.

Allsop, J., Baggott, R. and Jones, K. (2002) 'Health consumer groups and the national policy process', in A. Petersen and S. Henderson (eds) *Consuming health: The commodification of health care*, London: Routledge, pp 48-65.

Annandale, E. (2005) 'Missing connections: medical sociology and feminism', *Medical Sociology News*, vol 31, no 3, pp 35-52.

Annandale, E., Elston, M.A. and Prior, L. (eds) (2004) *Medical work, medical knowledge and health care*, Oxford: Blackwell.

AQUA (Institut für angewandte Qualitätsforschung) (2002) *Qualitätsindikatoren der AOK für Ärztenetze*, Göttingen: AQUA.

Atkinson, S. (2002) 'Political cultures, health systems and health policy', *Social Science and Medicine*, vol 55, pp 113-24.

Baggott, R. (2002) 'Regulatory politics, health professionals, and the public interest', in J. Allsop and M. Saks (eds) *Regulating the health professions*, London: Routledge, pp 31-46.

Baggott, R., Allsop, J. and Jones, K. (2005) *Speaking for patients and carers: Health consumer groups and the policy process*, Basingstoke: Palgrave.

BÄK (Bundesärztekammer) (1997) 'Tätigkeitsbericht '97', Unpublished report, Köln.

Bäringhausen, T. and Sauerborn, R. (2002) 'One hundred and eighteen years of the German health insurance system', *Social Science and Medicine*, vol 54, pp 1559-87.

Batterham, R., Southern, D., Appleby, N., Elsworth, G., Fabris, S., Dunt, D. and Young, D. (2002) 'Construction of GP integration model', *Social Science and Medicine*, vol 54, pp 1225-41.

BdA (Berufsverband der Arzt-, Zahnarzt- und Tierarzthelferinnen) (2003) 'Aktuelle Gehaltsstruktur in den Bundesländern; Zahlen und Fakten' (www.bda.de).

Beattie, A. (1991) 'Knowledge and control in health promotion: a test case for social policy and social theory', in J. Gabe, M. Calnan and M. Bury (eds) *The sociology of the health service*, London: Routledge, pp 162-202.

Beck, U. (1986) *Risikogesellschaft: Auf dem Weg in eine andere Moderne*, Frankfurt: Suhrkamp.

Bendelow, G., Carpenter, M., Vautier, C. and Williams, S. (eds) (2002) *Gender, health and healing: The public/private divide*, London: Routledge.

Benoit, C. (1999) 'Midwifery and health policy: equity, workers' rights and consumer choice in Canada and Sweden', in I. Hellberg, M. Saks and C. Benoit (eds) *Professional identities in transition: Cross-cultural dimensions*, Goteborg: Almquist & Wiksell International, pp 255-74.

Bertilsson, M. (1990) 'The welfare state, the professions and citizens', in R. Torstendahl and M. Burrage (eds) *The formation of professions: Knowledge, state and strategy*, London: Sage Publications, pp 114-33.

Best, A. and Glik, D. (2003) 'Research as a tool for integrative health service reform', in M. Kelner, B. Wellman, B. Pescosolido and M. Saks (eds) *Complementary and alternative medicine: Challenge and change*, London: Routledge, pp 239-54.

Bird, K. and Gottschall, K. (2004) 'Erosion of the male-breadwinner model? Female labour-market participation and family-leave policies in Germany', in H. Gottfried (ed) *Equity in the workplace: Gendering workplace policy analysis*, Lanham, MD: Lexington Books, pp 281-303.

Bissell, P., May, C.R. and Noyce, P.R. (2004) 'From compliance to concordance: barriers to accomplishing a re-framed model of health care interactions', *Social Science and Medicine*, vol 58, pp 851-62.

Blank, R.H. and Burau, V. (2004) *Comparative health policy*, Houndmills: Palgrave.

Blättel-Mink, B. and Kramer, C. (2006: forthcoming) 'Frauen im Arztberuf', in Institut für Länderkunde (eds) *Arbeit und Lebensstandard, Nationalatlas Bundesrepublik Deutschland*, Bd 7, Heidelberg: Springer.

Blättel-Mink, B. and Kuhlmann, E. (2003) 'Health professions, gender and society: introduction and outlook', *International Journal of Sociology and Social Policy*, vol 23, no 4/5, pp 1-21.

BLK (Bund-Länder-Kommission) (2004) *Frauen in der Medizin: Ausbildung und berufliche Situation von Medizinerinnen*, Bonn: BLK für Bildungsplanung und Forschungsförderung.

Blumenthal, D. (1996) 'Quality of care – what is it?', *New England Journal of Medicine*, vol 335, pp 891-94.

BMA (British Medical Association) (2004) 'Trust in doctors at its highest for twenty years, poll shows' (www.bma.org.uk).

BMG (Bundesministerium für Gesundheit) (2002) (www.bmgesundheit.de).

BMJ (British Medical Journal) (2006) 'Editorial. New directions for NHS community services', *BMJ*, vol 332, pp 315-16.

Bode, I. (2003) 'Multireferenzialität und Marktorientierung? Krankenkassen als hybride Organisationen im Wandel', *Zeitschrift für Soziologie*, vol 32, no 5, pp 435-53.

Bottomore, T. (1992) 'Forty years on', in T.H. Marshall and T. Bottomore (eds) *Citizenship and social class*, London: Pluto, pp 55-96.

Bourgeault, I.L. (2005) 'Rationalization of health care and female professional projects', *Knowledge, Work & Society*, vol 3, no 1, pp 25-52.

Bourgeault, I.L. and Fynes, M. (1997) 'Integrating lay and nurse-midwifery into the US and Canadian health care systems', *Social Science and Medicine*, vol 44, pp 1051-63.

Bourgeault, I.L., Benoit, C. and Davies-Floyd, R. (eds) (2004) *Reconceiving midwifery*, Kingston/Montreal: McGill Queen's University Press.

Braun, B. and Schnee, M. (2002) 'Vertrauen bei der Wahrnehmung und Bewertung von Akteuren, Institutionen und Eigenschaften des Gesundheitswesens', in J. Böcken, B. Braun and M. Schnee (eds) *Gesundheitsmonitor 2002*, Gütersloh: Bertelsmann, pp 173-87.

Braun, B., Calnan, M., Groenewegen, P., Schee, E. van der and Schnee, M. (2003) 'Zeitlicher und internationaler Vergleich des Vertrauens in Akteure, Institutionen und Eigenschaften des Gesundheitswesens', in J. Böcken, B. Braun and M. Schnee (eds) *Gesundheitsmonitor 2003*, Gütersloh: Bertelsmann, pp 136-68.

Brechtel, T. (2001) 'Ärztliche Interessenpolitik und Gesundheitsreform: Die Zufriedenheit niedergelassener Ärzte mit den Berufsverbänden vor und nach dem Gesundheitsstrukturgesetz', *Zeitschrift für Gesundheitswissenschaften*, vol 9, no 3, pp 273-88.

Broadbent, J. (1998) 'Practice nurses and effects on the new general practitioner contract in the British NHS: the advent of a professional project?', *Social Science and Medicine*, vol 47, pp 497-506.

Burau, V. (1999) 'The politics of internal boundaries: a comparative analysis of community nursing in Britain and Germany: some preliminary observations', in I. Hellberg, M. Saks and C. Benoit (eds) *Professional identities in transition: Cross-cultural dimensions*, Goteborg: Almquist & Wiksell International, pp 239-53.

Burau, V. (2005) 'Comparing professions through actor-based governance: community nursing in Britain and Germany', *Sociology of Health and Illness*, vol 27, pp 114-37.

Burau, V., Henriksson, L. and Wrede, S. (2004) 'Comparing professional groups: towards a context sensitive analysis', *Knowledge, Work & Society*, vol 2, no 2, pp 49-68.

Burrage, M. and Thorstendahl, R. (eds) (1990) *Professions in theory and history*, London: Sage Publications.

Busse, R. and Schlette, S. (eds) (2004) *Gesundheitspolitik in Industrieländern*, Gütersloh: Bertelsmann.

BWHBC (Boston Women's Health Book Collective) (1971) *Our bodies, ourselves*, New York, NY: Simon and Schuster.

Calnan, M.W. and Sanford, E. (2004) 'Public trust in health care: the system or the doctor?', *Quality and Safety in Health Care*, vol 13, pp 92-7.

Campbell, S.M., Roland, M.O. and Buetow, S.A. (2000) 'Defining quality of care', *Social Science and Medicine*, vol 51, pp 1611-25.

Clarke, J. (2004) *Changing welfare, changing states: New directions in social policy*, London: Sage Publications.

Clarke, J. (2005) 'Reconstituting Europe: governing a European people?', in J. Newman (ed) *Remaking governance*, Bristol: The Policy Press, pp 17-37.

Clarke, J. and Newman, J. (1997) *The managerial state*, London: Sage Publications.

Clarke, J., Smith, N. and Vidler, E. (2005) 'Consumerism and the reform of public services: inequalities and instabilities', in M. Powell, K. Clarke and L. Bauld (eds) *Social Policy Review 17*, Bristol: The Policy Press, pp 167-82.

Coburn, D. (1993) 'State authority, medical dominance, and trends in the regulation of the health professions: the Ontario case', *Social Science and Medicine*, vol 37, pp 841-50.

Coburn, D. (1999) 'Professions in transition: globalisation, neo-liberalism and the decline of medical power', in I. Hellberg, M. Saks and C. Benoit (eds) *Professional identities in transition: Cross-cultural dimensions*, Goteborg: Almquist & Wiksell International, pp 139-56.

Cochrane, A.L. (1972) *Effectiveness and efficiency: Random reflections on health services*, Abingdon: Burgess & Son.

Coleman, J.S. (1990) *The foundation of social theory*, CAMbridge, MA: Belknap Press.

Commission of the European Countries (2004) *Modernising social protection for the development of high-quality, accessible and sustainable health care and long-term care: Support for the national strategies using the 'Open Method of Coordination'*, Brussels, 20.04.2004, COM (2004) 304 final.

Coulson, A. (ed) (1998a) *Trust and contracts: Relationships in local government, health and social services*, Bristol: The Policy Press.

Coulson, A. (1998b) 'Trust: the foundation of public sector management', in A. Coulson (ed) *Trust and contracts: Relationships in local government, health and social services*, Bristol: The Policy Press, pp 3-8.

Currell, W., Wainwright, P. and Urquhart, C. (2002) 'Nursing record systems: effects on nursing practice and health care outcomes', *The Cochrane Library*, issue 2/2002.

Dahle, R. (2003) 'Shifting boundaries and negotiations on knowledge: interprofessional conflicts between nurses and nursing assistants in Norway', *International Journal of Sociology and Social Policy*, vol 23, no 4/5, pp 139-58.

Dahle, R. (2006: forthcoming) 'Temporary nurses: a gendered, flexible labour force in the Norwegian welfare state', *Knowledge, Work & Society*, vol 4, no 1.

Dale, J., Crouch, R. and Lloyd, D. (1998) 'Primary care: nurse-led telephone triage and advice out-of-hours', *Nursing Standard*, vol 12, no 47, pp 41-5.

Davies, C. (1996) 'The sociology of the professions and the profession of gender', *Sociology*, vol 30, no 4, pp 661-78.

Davies, C. (2002a) 'What about the girl next door? Gender and the politics of self-regulation', in G. Bendelow, M. Carpenter, C. Vautier and S. Williams (eds) *Gender, health and healing: The public/private divide*, London: Routledge, pp 91-107.

Davies, C. (2002b) 'Registering a difference: changes in the regulation of nursing', in J. Allsop and M. Saks (eds) *Regulating the health professions*, London: Routledge, pp 94-107.

Davies, C. (2003) 'Introduction: a new workforce in the making?', in C. Davies (ed) *The future health workforce*, Houndmills: Palgrave, pp 1-13.

Davies, C., Wetherell, M., Barnett, E. and Seymour-Smith, S. (2005) *Opening the box: Evaluating the citizen council of NICE*, Milton Keynes: The Open University, Report prepared for the National Co-ordinating Centre for Research Methodology, NHS Research and Development Programme.

Dean, K. (2004) 'The role of methods in maintaining orthodox beliefs in health research', *Social Science and Medicine*, vol 58, pp 675-85.

Dean, M. (1999) *Governmentality: Power and rule in modern society*, London: Sage Publications.

Delhey, J. and Newton, K. (2003) 'Who trusts? The origins of social trust in seven countries', *European Societies*, vol 5, no 2, pp 93-137.

Dent, M. (2003) *Remodelling hospitals and health professions in Europe*, Houndmills: Palgrave.

Deppe, H.-U. (2000) *Zur sozialen Anatomie des Gesundheitssystems: Neoliberalismus und Gesundheitspolitik in Deutschland*, Frankfurt: VAS.

Di Luzio, G. (2004) 'The irresistible decline of the medical profession? An empirical investigation of its autonomy and economic situation in the changing German welfare state', *German Politics*, vol 13, no 3, pp 419-38.

Dixon, A., Riesberg, A., Weinbrenner, S., Saka, O., Le Grand, J. and Busse, R. (2003) *Complementary and alternative medicine in the UK and Germany – Research and evidence on supply and demand*, Working Paper, Ango-German Foundation for the Study of Industrial Society (www.agf.org.uk).

Dobrow, M.J., Goel, V. and Upshur, R.E.G. (2004) 'Evidence-based health policy: context and utilisation', *Social Science and Medicine*, vol 58, pp 207-17.

Döhler, M. (1995) 'The state as architect of political order: policy dynamics in German health care', *Governance: An International Journal of Policy and Administration*, vol 8, no 3, pp 380-404.

Donabedian, A. (1988) 'The quality of care: how can it be assessed?', *Journal of the American Medical Association*, vol 260, pp 1743-8.

Donaldson, M.S., Yordy, K.D., Lohr, K.N. and Vanselow, N.A. (1996) *Primary care: America's health in a new era*, Washington, DC: National Academy Press.

Douglas, M. (1991) *Wie Institutionen denken*, Frankfurt: Suhrkamp.

Dowell, T. and Neal, R. (2000) 'Vision and change in primary care: past, present and future', in P. Tovey (ed) *Contemporary primary care: The challenges of change*, Milton Keynes: Open University Press, pp 9-25.

Dubois, C.-A., McKee, M. and Nolte, E. (eds) (2006) *Human resources for health in Europe*, Buckingham: Open University Press.

DuGay, P. and Salaman, G. (1992) 'The cult(ure) of the customer', *Journal of Management Studies*, vol 29, no 5, pp 615-33.

Durkheim, E. (1992 [1950]) *Professional ethics and civic morals*, London: Routledge.

Eckman, A.K. (1998) 'Beyond the Yentl syndrome: making women visible in the post-1990s women's health discourse', in P. Treichler, L. Cartwright and C. Penley (eds) *The visible woman*, New York, NY: New York University Press, pp 130-68.

Economist, The (2005) 'Rich countries everywhere are struggling to finance health care', 18 August (www.economist.com/world/Europe/displayStory.cfm?story_id=4293317).

Elston, S. and Holloway, I. (2001) 'The impact of recent primary care reforms in the UK on interprofessional working in primary care centres', *Journal of Interprofessional Care*, vol 15, pp 19-27.

Esping-Andersen, G. (ed) (1996) *Welfare states in transition*, London: Sage Publications.

Etzioni, A. (ed) (1969) *The semi-professions and their organization: Teachers, nurses, social workers*, New York, NY: Free Press.

European Observatory on Health Care Systems (2000) 'Health care systems in transition: Germany' (www.euro.who.int/document/e68952.pdf).

EUROPEP (European Working Party in Quality in Family Practice) (2002) 'The EUROPEP instrument' (www.swiss.pep.ch/pages/EUROPEP.html).

Evetts, J. (1999) 'Professions: changes and continuities', *International Review of Sociology*, vol 9, pp 75-85.

Evetts, J (2003) 'The construction of professionalism in new and existing contexts: promoting and facilitating occupational change', *International Journal of Sociology and Social Policy*, vol 23, no 4/5, pp 23-38.

Evetts, J. (2006a) 'The sociology of professional groups: new directions', *Current Sociology*, vol 54, no 1, pp 133-43.

Evetts, J. (2006b: forthcoming) 'Introduction: professions, trust and knowledge', *Current Sociology*, vol 54, no 4.

Exworthy, M., Wilkinson, E.K., McColl, A., Moore, M., Roderick, P., Smith, H. and Gabbay, J. (2003) 'The role of performance indicators in changing the autonomy of the general practice profession in the UK', *Social Science and Medicine*, vol 56, pp 1493-504.

Flood, A.B. (2004) 'Making evidence-based decisions in health: (or more importantly) using evidence when the case doesn't quite fit', *Women's Health Issues*, vol 14, pp 3-6.

Flynn, R. (2004) 'Soft bureaucracy, governmentality and clinical governance: theoretical approaches to emergent policy', in A. Grey and S. Harrison (eds) *Medical governance: Theory and practice*, Buckingham: Open University Press, pp 11-26.

Foucault, M. (1979) 'On governmentality', *Ideology and Consciousness*, vol 6, pp 5-22.

Fougere, G. (2001) 'Transforming health sectors: new logics of organizing in the New Zealand health system', *Social Science and Medicine*, vol 52, pp 1233-42.

Fournier, V. (1999) 'The appeal to "professionalism" as a disciplinary mechanism', *Sociological Review*, vol 47, no 2, pp 280-307.

Fournier, V. (2000) 'Boundary work and the (un)making of the professions', in N. Malin (ed) *Professionalism, boundaries and the workplace*, London: Routledge, pp 67-86.

Fox, R.C. (2002) 'Medical uncertainty revisited', in G. Bendelow, M. Carpenter, C. Vautier and S. Williams (eds) *Gender, health and healing: The public/private divide*, London: Routledge, pp 236-54.

Freeman, R. (2000) *The politics of health in Europe*, Manchester: Manchester University Press.

Freidson, E. (1986) *Professional powers: A study of formal knowledge*, Chicago, IL: Chicago University Press.

Freidson, E. (2001) *Professionalism: The third logic*, Oxford: Polity Press.

Fulop, N., Protopsalis, G., King, A., Allen, P., Hutchings, A. and Normand, C. (2005) 'Changing organisations: a study of the context and processes of mergers of health care providers in England', *Social Science and Medicine*, vol 60, pp 119-30.

Gabe, J. and Calnan, M. (2000) 'Health care and consumption', in S. Williams, J. Gabe and M. Calnan (eds) *Health, medicine and society: Key theories, future agendas*, London: Routledge, pp 255-73.

Gallagher, M., Huddart, T. and Henderson, B. (1998) 'Telephone triage of acute illness by a practice nurse in general practice: outcome of care', *British Journal of General Practice*, vol 48, April, pp 1141-5.

Gartner, A. and Riessman, F. (1978) *Der aktive Konsument in der Dienstleistungsgesellschaft*, Frankfurt: Suhrkamp.

GBE (Gesundheitsbericht für Deutschland) (1998a) 'Erwerbstätige im Gesundheitswesen' (www.gbe-bund.de).

GBE (1998b) 'Leistungen nichtärztlicher medizinischer Berufe, Kapitel 7.6' (www.gbe-bund.de).

GBE (2002) (www.gbe-bund.de).

GBE (2005) (www.gbe-bund.de).

Gerrish, K. (1999) 'Teamwork in primary care: an evaluation of the contribution of integrated nursing teams', *Health and Social Care in the Community*, vol 7, no 5, pp 367-75.

Gerst, T., Rieser, S. and Stüwe, H. (2005) 'Interview mit Dr jur Rainer Daubenbüchel', *Deutsches Ärzteblatt*, vol 102, p A-91.

Giddens, A. (1991) *Modernity and self-identity: Self and society in the late modern age*, CAMbridge: Polity Press.

Giddens, A. (1998) *The third way: The renewal of social democracy*, CAMbridge: Polity Press.

Giddens, A., Beck, U. and Lash, S. (1994) *Reflexive modernisation*, CAMbridge: Polity Press.

Gillam, S. (2003) 'The future of the general practitioner', in C. Davies (ed) *The future health workforce*, Houndmills: Palgrave, pp 181-98.

Gilson, L. (2003) 'Trust and the development of health care as a social institution', *Social Science and Medicine*, vol 56, pp 1453-68.

Glaeske, G., Lauterbach, K.W., Rürup, B. and Wasem, J. (2001) *Weichenstellung für die Zukunft – Elemente einer neuen Gesundheitspolitik*, Berlin: Gutachten für die Friedrich-Ebert-Stiftung.

Gonen, J.S. (1999a) 'Quality in women's health: taking the measure of managed care', *Women's Health Issues*, vol 9, no 2, Suppl 1, pp 79S-88S.

Gonen, J.S. (1999b) 'Women's primary care in managed care: clinical and provider issues', *Women's Health Issues*, vol 9, no 2, Suppl 1, pp 5S-14S.

Gonen, J.S. (1999c) 'Health plans and purchasers: managing women's primary care', *Women's Health Issues*, vol 9, no 2, Suppl 1, pp 15S-25S.

Goni, S. (1999) 'An analysis of the effectiveness of Spanish primary care teams', *Health Policy*, vol 48, pp 107-17.

Goudge, J. and Gilson, L. (2005) 'How can trust be investigated? Drawing lessons from past experience', *Social Science and Medicine*, vol 61, pp 1439-51.

Gray, A. and Harrison, S. (eds) (2004) *Governing medicine: Theory and practice*, Buckingham: Open University Press.

Greer, A.L. (1998) 'The end of splendid isolation: tensions between science and practice', in C. Meyer (ed) *Expert witnessing: Explaining and understanding science*, Boca Raton: CRL Press, pp 51-65.

Greß, S., Gildemeister, S. and Wasem, J. (2004) 'The social transformation of American medicine: a comparative view from Germany', *Journal of Health Politics, Policy and Law*, vol 29, pp 679-99.

Grol, R., Baker, R. and Moss, F. (2002) 'Quality improvement research: understanding the science of change in health care', *Quality and Safety in Health Care*, vol 11, pp 110-11.

Hall, D. and Soskice, D. (eds) (2001) *Varieties of capitalism*, Oxford: Oxford University Press.

Haraway, D.J. (1991) *Simians, cyborgs, and women: The reinvention of nature*, New York, NY: Routledge.

Haraway, D.J. (1997) *Modest_Witness@second_millennium. FemaleMan© _meets_oncomouse^{TM}*, New York, NY: Routledge.

Harrison, S. (1998) 'The politics of evidence-based medicine in the United Kingdom', *Policy & Politics*, vol 26, no 1, pp 15-31.

Harrison, S. (2004) 'Medicine and management: autonomy and authority in the national health service', in A. Grey and S. Harrison (eds) *Medical governance: Theory and practice*, Buckingham: Open University Press, pp 51-9.

Harrison, S. and Ahmad, W.I.U. (2000) 'Medical autonomy and the UK state 1975 to 2025', *Sociology*, vol 34, no 1, pp 129-46.

Harrison, S. and Mort, M. (1998) 'Which champions, which people? Public and user involvement in health care as a technology of legitimation', *Social Policy and Administration*, vol 32, pp 60-70.

Harrison, S. and Smith, C. (2004) 'Trust and moral motivation: redundant resources in health and social care?', *Policy & Politics*, vol 32, no 3, pp 371-86.

Häussler, B., Glaeske, G. and Gothe, H. (2001) 'Unbeantwortete Fragen zum Disease-Management', *Arbeit und Sozialpolitik*, vol 9, no 10, pp 35-7.

Healy, B. (1991) 'The yentle syndrome', *New England Journal of Medicine*, vol 325, pp 274-6.

HEDIS (Health Plan Employer Data and Information Set) (2002) (www.ncqa.org/programs/HEDIS/html).

Heiligers, P.J.M. and Hingstman, L. (2000) 'Career preferences and the work-family balance in medicine: differences among medical specialists', *Social Science and Medicine*, vol 50, pp 1235-46.

Hellberg, I. (1999) 'Altruism and utility: two logics of professional action', in I. Hellberg, M. Saks and C. Benoit (eds) *Professional identities in transition: Cross-cultural dimensions*, Goteborg: Almquist & Wiksell International, pp 27-41.

Hellberg, I., Saks, M. and Benoit, C. (eds) (1999) *Professional identities in transition: Cross-cultural dimensions*, Goteborg: Almquist & Wiksell International.

Higgs, P. (1998) 'Risk, governmentality and the reconceptualization of citizenship', in G. SCAMbler and P. Higgs (eds) *Modernity, medicine and health*, New York, NY: Routledge, pp 186-97.

Hill, P.S. (2002) 'The rhetorics of sector-wide approaches for health development', *Social Science and Medicine*, vol 54, pp 1725-37.

Hindress, B. (1993) 'Citizenship in the modern west', in B.S. Turner (ed) *Citizenship and social theory*, London: Sage Publications, pp 19-35.

Hoffman, E., Maraldo, P., Coons, H.L. and Johnson, K. (1997) 'The women-centred health care team: integrating perspectives from managed care: women's health, and the health professional workforce', *Women's Health Issues*, vol 7, no 6, pp 362-74.

Hughes, D. and Griffiths, L. (1999) 'On penalties and the patient's charter: centralism versus de-centralised governance in the NHS', *Sociology of Health and Illness*, vol 21, pp 71-94.

Hüter-Becker, A. (1998) 'Von der Heilgymnastik zur Physiothearapie', *Krankengymnastik*, vol 50, no 3, pp 456-66.

Hüter-Becker, A. (1999) '50 Jahre Berufspolitik: 1949-1999', *Krankengymnastik*, vol 51, no 10, pp 1679-86.

Isfort, J., Floer, B. and Butzlaff, M. (2004) 'Shared decision-making: partizipative Entscheidungsfindung auf dem Weg in die Praxis', in J. Böcken, B. Braun and M. Schnee (eds) *Gesundheitsmonitor 2004*, Gütersloh: Bertelsmann, pp 88-100.

Isin, E.F. and Turner, B.S. (2002) 'Citizenship studies: an introduction', in E.F. Isin and B.S. Turner (eds) *Handbook of citizenship studies*, London: Sage Publications, pp 1-10.

Jenkins-Clarke, S., Carr-Hill, R. and Dixon, P. (1998) 'Teams and seams: skill mix in primary care', *Nursing and Health Care Management Issues*, vol 28, no 5, pp 1120-6.

Johnson, T. (1972) *Professions and power*, London: Macmillan.

Johnson, T. (1995) 'Governmentality and the institutionalization of expertise', in T. Johnson, G. Larkin and M. Saks (eds) *Health professions and the state in Europe*, London, Routledge, pp 7-24.

Johnson, T., Larkin, G. and Saks, M. (eds) (1995) *Health professions and the state in Europe*, London: Routledge.

Kaufmann, X.-F. (1997) *Herausforderungen des Sozialstaates*, Frankfurt: Suhrkamp.

Kaukewitsch, D. (2002) 'Jobmaschine Gesundheitswesen', *Praxisnah, Journal des BdA*, no 10, p 5.

Kaukewitsch, D. (2003) 'Arbeitslosigkeit seit vier Jahren rückläufig', *Praxisnah, Journal des BdA*, no 1/2, pp 8-9.

KBV (Kassenärztliche Bundesvereinigung) (2000) *Grunddaten zur Vetragsärztlichen Versorgung in der Bundesrepublik Deutschland 2000*, Köln: KBV Referat Bedarfsplanung, Bundesarztregister und Datenaustausch.

KBV (2002a) 'Modellvorhaben und Strukturverträge' (www.kbv.de).

KBV (2002b) 'Jahresbericht', Köln: KBV.

Kelner, M., Wellman, B., Boon, H. and Welsh, S. (2004) 'Responses of established healthcare to the professionalization of complementary and alternative medicine in Ontario', *Social Science and Medicine*, vol 59, pp 915-30.

Kelner, M., Wellman, B., Pescosolido, B. and Saks, M. (eds) (2003) *Complementary and alternative medicine: Challenge and change*, London: Routledge.

Kerssens, J.F., Bensing, J.M. and Andela, M.G. (1997) 'Patient preference for genders of health professionals', *Social Science and Medicine*, vol 44, pp 1531-40.

Kirkpatrick, I., Ackroyd, S. and Walker, R. (2005) *The new managerialism and public service professions: Change in health, social services and housing*, Houndmills: Palgrave.

Knorr-Cetina, K. (1981) *The transformation of knowledge: An essay on constructionist and contextual nature of science*, Oxford: Pergamon.

Koninck, M. de, Bergeron, P. and Bourbannais, R. (1997) 'Women physicians in Quebec', *Social Science and Medicine*, vol 44, pp 1825-32.

Kremer, M. (2005) 'The duty to choose: free choice in the Dutch welfare state', Paper presented to the 'Reinventing the Public' Conference, Milton Keynes, 15-17 April.

Krimmel, L. (2000) 'Gesetzliche Krankenversicherung: Stiller Abschied vom "medizinisch Notwendigen"', *Deutsches Ärzteblatt*, vol 97, no 16, p A-1052.

Krüger, H. (2001) 'Pflegeberufe in der Dienstleistungsgesellschaft – Zwang zur bildungspolitischen Gestaltung', in P. Kiesel, H. Krüger, G. Piechotta, H. Remmers and J. Taubert (eds) *Pflege lehren – Pflege managen: Eine Bilanzierung innovativer Ansätze*, Frankfurt: Mabuse, pp 21-42.

Kuhlmann, E. (1998) 'Zwischen zwei Mahlsteinen: Ergebnisse einer empirischen Studie zur Verteilung knapper medizinischer Ressourcen', in G. Feuerstein and E. Kuhlmann (eds) *Rationierung im Gesundheitswesen*, Wiesbaden: Ullstein Medical, pp 11-80.

Kuhlmann, E. (1999) 'Aufklärung im Dienst der Ressourcenallokation? Eine empirische Studie zur ärztlichen Informationspolitik', in G. Feuerstein and E. Kuhlmann (eds) *Neopaternalistische Medizin*, Bern: Hans Huber, pp 37-94.

Kuhlmann, E. (2001) 'The rise of German dental professionalism as a gendered project: how scientific progress and health policy evoked change in gender relations, 1850-1919', *Medical History*, vol 45, pp 443-60.

Kuhlmann, E. (2002) 'Humangenetik und Geschlecht: Formationen zwischen Hegemonie und Autonomiekonstrukten', in E. Kuhlmann and R. Kollek (eds) *Konfiguration des Menschen: Biowissenschaften als Arena der Geschlechterpolitik*, Opladen: Leske + Budrich, pp 61-77.

Kuhlmann, E. (2003) 'Gender differences, gender hierarchies and professions: an embedded approach to the German dental profession', *International Journal of Sociology and Social Policy*, vol 23, no 4/5, pp 80-96.

Kuhlmann, E. (2004) 'Post-modern times for professions – the fall of the "ideal professional" and its challenges to theory', *Knowledge, Work and Society*, vol 2, no 2, pp 69-89.

Kuhlmann, E. (2006a: forthcoming) 'Towards "citizen professionals": new patterns of professionalism in health care in Germany', *Knowledge, Work & Society*, vol 4, no 1.

Kuhlmann, E. (2006b) 'Traces of doubt and sources of trust – health professions in an uncertain society', *Current Sociology*, vol 54, no 4, pp 607-20.

Kuhlmann, E. and Babitsch, B. (2002) 'Bodies, health, gender – bridging feminist theories and women's health', *Women's Studies International Forum*, vol 25, pp 433-42.

Kuhlmann, E. and Kolip, P. (2005) *Gender und public health: Orientierungen für Forschung, Praxis und Politik*, Weinheim: Juventa.

Kuhlmann, E., Werner, B. and Wilm, B. (1997) *Analyse und Identifikation von Qualifikationsanforderungen und Qualifizierungsfeldern für nicht-ärztliche Beschäftige im Gesundheitssektor*, Expertise für das Ministerium für Gesundheiteit, Arbeit und Soziales Nordrhein-Westfalen, Bielefeld: Institut für Pflegewissenschaft.

Kühn, H. (1997) *Managed care: Medizin zwischen kommerzieller Bürokratie und integrierter Versorgung*, Discussion Paper P97-102, Berlin: Wissenschaftszentrum Berlin für Sozialforschung.

Kühn, H. (2001) *Integration der medizinischen Versorgung in regionaler Perspektive,* Discussion Paper P01-202, Berlin: Wissenschaftszentrum Berlin für Sozialforschung.

Kunstmann, W. and Butzlaff, M. (2004) 'Ärztliche Therapiefreiheit und Fortbildungspflicht – ein Widerspruch? Perspektiven und Einschätzungen aus der Ärzteschaft', in J. Böcken, B. Braun and M. Schnee (eds) *Gesundheitsmonitor 2004,* Gütersloh: Bertelsmann, pp 75-87.

Larson, M.S. (1977) *The rise of professionalism,* Berkeley, CA: University of California Press.

Larson, M.S. (1979) 'Professionalism: rise and fall', *International Journal of Health Services,* vol 9, no 4, pp 607-27.

Larson, M.S. (1990) 'In the matter of experts and professionals, or how impossible it is to leave nothing unsaid', in R. Thorstendahl and M. Burrage (eds) *Knowledge, state and strategy,* London: Sage Publications, pp 24-50.

Latour, B. and Woolgar, S. (1986) *Laboratory life: The social construction of scientific facts,* Princeton, NJ: Princeton University Press.

Leca, J. (1992) 'Questions on citizenship', in C. Mouffe (ed) *Dimensions of radical democracy,* London: Verso, pp 17-32.

Lee, R.G. and Garvin, T. (2003) 'Moving from information transfer to information exchange', *Social Science and Medicine,* vol 56, pp 449-64.

Leiter, M.P., Harvie, P. and Frizzell, C. (1998) 'The correspondence of patient-satisfaction and nurse burnout', *Social Science and Medicine,* vol 47, pp 1611-17.

Lewis, J. (2002) 'Gender and welfare state change', *European Societies,* vol 4, no 4, pp 331-57.

Light, D.W. (1995) 'Countervailing powers: a framework for professions in transition', in T. Johnson, G. Larkin and M. Saks (eds) *Health professions and the state in Europe,* London: Routledge, pp 7-24.

Light, D.W. (1997) 'The rhetorics and realities of community health care: the limits of countervailing powers to meet the health care needs of the twenty-first century', *Journal of Health Politics, Policy and Law,* vol 22, pp 104-45.

Light, D.W. (2001) 'Comparative institutional response to economic policy, managed competition and governmentality', *Social Science and Medicine,* vol 52, pp 1167-81.

Lindbladh, E., Lyttkens, C.H., Hanson, B.S. and Östergren, P.-O. (1998) 'Equity is out of fashion? An essay on autonomy and health policy in the individualized society', *Social Science and Medicine,* vol 46, pp 1017-25.

Lingenfelder, M. and Kronhardt, M. (2003) 'Erfolgsfaktoren medizinischer Versorgungsnetze', in H. Pfaff, M. Schrappe, K.W. Lauterbach, U. Engelmann and H. Halber (eds) *Gesundheitsversorgung und Disease Management*, Bern: Hans Huber, pp 109-16.

Löyttyniemi, V. (2001) 'Doctors drifting: autonomy and career uncertainty in young physicians' stories', *Social Science and Medicine*, vol 52, pp 227-37.

Lucas, K. and Bickler, G. (2000) 'Altogether now? Professional differences in the priorities of primary care groups', *Journal of Public Health Medicine*, vol 22, no 2, pp 211-15.

Lupton, D. (1997) 'Consumerism, reflexivity and the medical encounter', *Social Science and Medicine*, vol 45, pp 373-81.

Macdonald, K. (1995) *The sociology of the professions*, London: Sage Publications.

McClelland, C.E. (1990) 'Escape from freedom? Reflections on German professionalization, 1870-1933', in R. Torstendahl and M. Burrage (eds) *The formation of professions*, London: Sage Publications, pp 97-114.

McConnell, C.R. (2002) 'The health care professional as a manager: finding the critical balance in a dual role', *Health Care Manager*, vol 20, no 3, pp 1-10.

McDonald, R. and Harrison, S. (2004) 'The micropolitics of clinical guidelines: an empirical study', *Policy & Politics*, vol 13, pp 223-39.

McKee, M., Dubois, C.-A. and Sibbard, B. (2006) 'Changing professional boundaries', in C.-A. Dubois, M. McKee and E. Nolte (eds) *Human resources for health in Europe*, Buckingham: Open University Press, pp 63-78.

McKinley, E.D., Thompson, J.W., Briefer-French, J., Wilcox, L.S., Weisman, C.S. and Andrews, W.C. (2001) 'Performance indicators in women's health: incorporating women's health in the Health Plan Employer Data and Information Set (HEDIS)', *Women's Health Issues*, vol 12, pp 46-58.

Mclaughlin, J. and Webster, A. (1998) 'Rationalising knowledge: IT systems, professional identities and power', *The Sociological Review*, vol 46, no 4, pp 781-802.

Marburger Bund (2002) *Ärztinnen: Situation, Probleme, Chancen*, Köln: Marburger Bund.

Marshall, T.H. (1992 [1950]) 'Citizenship and social class', in T.H. Marshall and T. Bottomore (eds) *Citizenship and social class*, London: Pluto, pp 3-51.

Marstedt, G. (2003) 'Auf der Suche nach gesundheitlicher Information und Beratung: Befunde zum Wandel der Patientenrolle', in J. Böcken, B. Braun and M. Schnee (eds) *Gesundheitsmonitor 2003*, Gütersloh: Bertelsmann, pp 117-35.

Martin, E. (1994) *Flexible bodies: Tracking immunity in American culture – from the days of polio to the age of AIDS*, Boston, MA: Beacon Press.

Mechanic, D. (1991) 'Sources of countervailing power in medicine', *Journal of Health Politics, Policy and Law*, vol 16, no 3, pp 485-98.

Mechanic, D. (1998) 'The functions and limitations of trust in the provision of medical care', *Journal of Health Politics, Policy and Law*, vol 23, no 4, pp 661-86.

Mechanic, D. and Meyer, S. (2000) 'Concepts of trust among patients with serious illness', *Social Science and Medicine*, vol 51, pp 657-68.

Menarguez Puche, J.F. and Saturno Hernandez, P.J. (1999) 'Description del clima organizacional en equipos de atencion primaria de una communidad autonoma', *Aten Primaria*, vol 23, no 5, pp 280-8.

Miller, P. and Rose, N. (1990) 'Governing economic life', *Economy and Society*, vol 19, no 1, pp 1-31.

Molyneux, J. (2001) 'Interprofessional teamworking: what makes teams work well?', *Journal of Interprofessional Care*, vol 15, no 1, pp 29-35.

Moran, M. (1999) *Governing the health care state*, Manchester: Manchester University Press.

Moran, M. (2004) 'Governing doctors in the British regulatory state', in A. Grey and S. Harrison (eds) *Medical governance: Theory and practice*, Buckingham: Open University Press, pp 27-36.

Mundinger, M.O., Kane, R.L., Lenz, E.R., Totten, A.M., Tsai, W.-Y., Cleary, P.D., Friedewald, W.T., Siu, A.L. and Shelanski, M.L. (2000) 'Primary care outcomes in patients treated by nurse practitioners or physicians', *Journal of the American Medical Association*, vol 283, pp 59-68.

Nagel, R. (2002) 'Integrierte ambulante Versorgung und Vernetzung: Empirische Untersuchung zur Akzeptanz und Erwartungshaltung bei Ärzten und Patienten eines Ärztenetzes', unpublished Masters thesis, Bremen: Universität Bremen.

Nagel, R. (2004) 'Befragung der Bezirksstelle Münster II: Motive für oder gegen den Beitritt zu einem Ärztenetz', unpublished manuscript, Kompetenzzentrum Ärztliche Kooperationen der KVWL.

Nancarrow, S. and Borthwick, A. (2005) 'Dynamic professional boundaries in the healthcare workforce', *Sociology of Health & Illness*, vol 27, pp 897-919.

Newman, J. (1998) 'The dynamics of trust', in A. Coulson (ed) *Trust and contracts: Relationship in local government, health and social services*, Bristol: The Policy Press, pp 35-51.

Newman, J. (2001) *Modernising governance: New labour, policy and governance*, London: Sage Publications.

Newman, J. (ed) (2005a) *Remaking governance: People, politics and the public sphere*, Bristol: The Policy Press.

Newman, J. (2005b) 'Conclusion', in J. Newman (ed) *Remaking governance: People, politics and the public sphere*, Bristol: The Policy Press, pp 197-213.

Newman, J. and Kuhlmann, E. (2007: forthcoming) 'Consumers enter the political stage: modernisation of health care in Britain and Germany', *European Journal of Social Policy*, vol 17, no 2.

Newman, J. and Vidler, E. (2006: forthcoming) 'Discriminating consumers, responsible patients, empowered users: consumerism and the modernisation of health care', *Journal of Social Policy*.

NHS CRD (National Health Service Centre for Reviews and Dissemination) (1999) 'Getting evidence into practice', *Effective Health Care*, vol 5, no 1.

Oakley, A. (2000) *Experiments in knowing*, New York, NY: The New Press.

O'Cathain, A., Goode, J., Luff, D., Strangleman, T., Hanlon, G. and Greatbatch, D. (2005) 'Does NHS Direct empower patients?', *Social Science and Medicine*, vol 61, pp 1761-71.

Offe, C. (2003) 'Micro-aspects of democratic theory: what makes for the deliberative competence of citizens?', in C. Offe (ed) *Herausforderungen der Demokratie*, Frankfurt/New York, NY: CAMpus, pp 297-334.

Olgiati, V. (2003) 'Geopolitical constructionism: the challenge of Europe to the comparative sociology of professions', in L.G. Svensson and J. Evetts (eds) *Conceptual and comparative studies of continental and Anglo-American professions*, Goteborg: Goteborg University, pp 55-77.

Parry, N. and Parry, J. (1976) *The rise of the medical profession*, London: Croom Helm.

Parsons, T. (1949) 'The professions in the social structure', in T. Parsons, *Essays in sociological theory*, Glencoe, IL: Free Press.

Peckham, S. and Exworthy, M. (2003) *Primary care in the UK*, Basingstoke: Palgrave.

Perkin, H. (1989) *The rise of professional society*, London: Routledge.

Pfaff, H., Schrappe, M., Lauterbach, K.W., Engelmann, U. and Halber, M. (eds) (2003) *Gesundheitsversorgung und Disease Management*, Bern: Hans Huber.

Porter, T.M. (1995) *Trust in numbers: The pursuit of objectivity in science and public life*, Princeton, NJ: Princeton University Press.

Rafferty, A.M., Ball, J. and Aiken, L.H. (2001) 'Are teamwork and professional autonomy compatible, and do they result in improved hospital care?', *Quality in Health Care*, vol 10, Suppl II, pp 32-7.

Reich, M.R. (2002) 'Reshaping the state from above, from within, from below: implications for public health', *Social Science and Medicine*, vol 54, pp 1669-75.

Richards, A., Carley, J., Jenkins-Clarke, S. and Richards, D.A. (2000) 'Skill mix between nurses and doctors working in primary care-delegation or allocation: a review of the literature', *International Journal of Nursing Studies*, vol 37, pp 185-97.

Richardson, B. (1999) 'Professional development', *Physiotherapy*, vol 85, pp 461-7.

Richardson, G., Maynard, A., Cullum, N. and Kindig, D. (1998) 'Skill mix changes: substitution or service development?', *Health Policy*, vol 45, pp 119-32.

Richter, E.A. (2000) 'Arzthelferinnen – Wie soll das Berufsbild zukünftig aussehen?', *Deutsches Ärzteblatt*, vol 97, no 26, p C-1349.

Riska, E. (2001a) *Medical careers and feminist agendas: American, Scandinavian, and Russian women physicians*, New York, NY: Aldine de Gruyter.

Riska, E. (2001b) 'Towards gender balance: but will women physicians have an impact on medicine?', *Social Science and Medicine*, vol 52, pp 187-97.

Riska, E. and Wrede, S. (2003) 'The hardy nurse: a professional discourse on self-regulation and emotional control in a female profession', in L.G. Svensson and J. Evetts (eds) *Conceptual and comparative studies of continental and Anglo-American professions*, Goteborg: Goteborg University Press, pp 153-69.

Robelet, M. (2005) 'Health professions, networks and co-ordination in the French health care system', Paper presented to the 7th ESA Conference, session RN 'Sociology of Professions', 8-12 September, Torun, Poland.

Robinson, R. and Steiner, A. (1998) *Managed health care: US evidence and lessons for the National Health Service*, Buckingham: Open University Press.

Robra, B.-P. (2005) 'Qualitätstransparenz – von der Ebene der Individualmedizin zur Ebene des Gesundheitswesens', in J. Klauber, B.-P. Robra and H. Schellschmidt (eds) *KrankenhausReport 2005*, Stuttgart: Schattauer, pp 3-15.

Rose, N. (1999) *Powers of freedom*, CAMbridge: CAMbridge University Press.

Rosenbrock, R. and Gerlinger, T. (2004) *Gesundheitspolitik: Eine systematische Einführung*, Bern: Hans Huber.

Rosenthal, F. and Boxberg, E. (1997) *Handbuch für medizinische Fachberufe*, Münster: MBO Verlag.

Sackett, D.L., Richardson, W.S., Rosenberg, W. and Haynes, R.B. (1997) *Evidence-based medicine*, New York, NY: Churchill-Livingstone.

Saks, M. (1995) *Professions and the public interest: Medical power, altruism and alternative medicine*, London: Routledge.

Saks, M. (1999) 'Towards integrated health care: shifting professional interests and identities in Britain', in I. Hellberg, M. Saks and C. Benoit (eds) *Professional identities in transition: Cross-cultural dimensions*, Goteborg: Almquist & Wiksell International, pp 295-309.

Saks, M. (2003a) 'The limitations of the Ango-American sociology of the professions: a critique of the currently dominant neo-Weberian orthodoxy', *Knowledge, Work & Society*, vol 1, no 1, pp 11-31.

Saks, M. (2003b) *Orthodox and alternative medicine: Politics, professionalization and health care*, London: Sage Publications.

Saks, M. (2003c) 'Professionalization, politics and CAM', in M. Kelner, B. Wellman, B. Pescosolido and M. Saks (eds) *Complementary and alternative medicine: Challenge and change*, London: Routledge, pp 223-38.

Saks, M. and Kuhlmann, E. (eds) (2006: forthcoming) 'Professions, social inclusion and citizenship: challenge and change in European health systems', *Knowledge, Work and Society*, vol 4, no 1, special issue.

Saltman, R.B. (2002) 'Regulating incentives: the past and present role of the state in health care systems', *Social Science and Medicine*, vol 54, pp 1677-84.

Sandall, J., Bourgeault, I.L., Meyer, W.J. and Schücking, B.A. (2001) 'Deciding who cares', in R. de Vries, C. Benoit, E.R. Teijlingen and S. Wrede (eds) *Birth by design*, New York, NY: Routledge, pp 117-38.

Sarasin, P. (2001) *Reizbare Maschinen: Eine Geschichte des Körpers 1765-1914*, Frankfurt/Main: Suhrkamp.

Sauerland, D. (2001) 'The German strategy for quality improvement in health care: still to improve', *Health Policy*, vol 56, pp 127-47.

Savage, M. and Witz, A. (1992) *Gender and bureaucracy*, Oxford: Blackwell.

Schämann, A. (2002) 'Physiotherapieforschung im internationalen Vergleich', *Krankengymnastik – Zeitschrift für Physiotherapeuten*, vol 54, pp 1282-90.

Scharnetzky, E., Deitermann, B., Michel, C. and Glaeske, G. (2004) *GEK Heil- und Hilfsmittelreport 2004*, St Augustin: Asgard.

Scheibler, F., Janßen, C. and Pfaff, H. (2003) 'Shared decision making: Ein Überblick über die internationale Forschungsliteratur', *Sozial- und Präventivmedizin*, vol 48, pp 11-23.

Schepers, R.M.J. and Casparie, A.F. (1999) 'Medical quality assurance and professional identity in Belgium, the Netherlands and England', in I. Hellberg, M. Saks and C. Benoit (eds) *Professional identities in transition: Cross-cultural dimensions*, Goteborg: Almquist & Wiksell International, pp 121-37.

Schmacke, N. (2002) *Leitlinienorientierung, evidenzbasierte Versorgung und Vertrauen in die Medizin: Voraussetzungen für die Entwicklung von strukturierten Behandlungsprogrammen*, Bonn: AOK.

Schmacke, N. (2003) *Qualitätsindikatoren für Ärztenetze als Beitrag zur Innovation der medizinischen Versorgung*, Bonn: AOK.

Schmidt, I.K. and Svarstadt, B.L. (2002) 'Nurse-physician communication and quality of drug use in Swedish nursing homes', *Social Science and Medicine*, vol 54, pp 1767-77.

Schöffski, O. and Schulenburg, M. Graf von der (1997) 'Unintended effects of a cost-containment policy: results of a natural experiment in Germany', *Social Science and Medicine*, vol 45, pp 1537-9.

Schwartz, F.W. and Busse, R. (1997) 'Germany', in C. Ham (ed) *Health care reform: Learning from international experience*, Buckingham: Open University Press, pp 114-18.

Schwewior-Popp, S. (1994) *Krankengymnastik und Ergotherapie: Eine exemplarische Studie zur Entwicklung von Professionalisierungsprozessen und Ausbildung in den Berufen des Gesundheitswesens*, Idstein: Schulz-Kirschner Verlag.

Sharma, U. (2003) 'Medical pluralism and the future of CAM', in M. Kelner, B. Wellman, B. Pescosolido and M. Saks (eds) *Complementary and alternative medicine: Challenge and change*, London: Routledge, pp 211-22.

Sheaff, R., Mashall, M., Rogers, A., Roland, M., Sibbald, B. and Pickard, S. (2004) 'Governmentality by network in English primary healthcare', *Social Policy & Administration*, vol 38, no 1, pp 89-103.

Shine, K.I. (2000) 'Closing the gap in quality of health care for Americans', *Circulations*, vol 101, pp 2325-7.

Shine, K.I. (2002) 'Health care quality and how to achieve it', *Academic Medicine*, vol 77, pp 91-9.

Sicotte, C., D'Amour, D. and Moreault, M.-P. (2002) 'Interdisciplinary collaboration within Quebec community health care centres', *Social Science and Medicine*, vol 55, pp 991-1003.

Siim, B. (2000) *Gender and citizenship: Politics and agency in France, Britain and Denmark*, CAMbridge: CAMbridge University Press.

Simmel, G. (1950) *The sociology of Georg Simmel* (edited by K. Wolff), Glencoe, IL: Free Press.

Southern, D.M., Young, D., Dunt, D., Appleby, N.J. and Batterham, R.W. (2002) 'Integration of primary care services: perceptions of Australian general practitioners, non-general practitioner health service providers and consumers at the general practice-primary care interface', *Evaluation and Program Planning*, vol 25, pp 47-59.

Stacey, M. (1992) *Regulating British medicine: The General Medical Council*, Chichester: Wiley.

Stamer, M. (2002) *Qualität durch Vernetzung – Das Oldenburger Modellprojekt: Qualitätsverbesserung auf der Ebene des Care Managements*, Hannover: Zentrum für Qualitätsmanagement im Gesundheitswesen, Ärztekammer Niedersachsen.

Starfield, B. and Shi, L. (2002) 'Policy relevant determinants of health: an international perspective', *Health Policy*, vol 60, pp 201-18.

StatBA (Statistisches Bundesamt Deutschland) (2003a) 'Pressemitteilung', 24 April (www.destatis.de/presse/deutsch/pm2003/p1610095.htm).

StatBA (2003b) 'Gesundheit: Ausgaben und Personal 2001' (www.destatis.de).

StatBA (2004) 'Pressemitteilung', 4 March.

Stevenson, K., Baker, R., Farooqi, A., Sorrie, R. and Khunti, K. (2001) 'Features of primary health care teams associated with successful quality improvement of diabetes care', *Family Practice*, vol 18, no 1, pp 21-6.

Stillfried, D. Graf von (2000) 'Integrationsversorgung – Innovationspotenzial und Risiken', *Sozialer Fortschritt*, vol 49, no 8/9, pp 175-84.

Streich, W. (2003) 'Private Gesundheitsausgaben', *Gesundheitsmonitor, Newsletter der Bertelsmann Stiftung*, no 4 (www.healthpolicymonitor.org).

Sullivan, M. (2003) 'The new subjective medicine: taking the patient's point of view on health care and health', *Social Science and Medicine*, vol 56, pp 1595-604.

Svensson, L.G. and Evetts, J. (eds) (2003a) *Conceptual and comparative studies of continental and Anglo-American professions*, Goteborg: Goteborg University Press.

Svensson, L.G. and Evetts, J. (2003b) 'Introduction', in L.G. Svensson and J. Evetts (eds) *Conceptual and comparative studies of continental and Anglo-American professions*, Goteborg: Goteborg University Press, pp 5-17.

SVR (Sachverständigenrat im Gesundheitswesen, Advisory Council for Concerted Action in Health Care) (2000/01) *Appropriateness and efficiency*, Report summary, English version (www.svr-gesundheit.de/Gutachten/Gutacht00/Kurz-eng100.pdf).

SVR (2003) *Health care finance, user orientation and quality*, Report summary, English version (www.svr-gesundheit.de/Gutachten/Gutacht03/Kurz-eng103.pdf).

SVR (2005) *Koordination und Qualität im Gesundheitswesen* (www.svr-gesundheit.de/Gutachten/Gutacht05/Kurzfassung.pdf).

Theobald, H. (2003) 'Care for the elderly: welfare system, professionalization and the question of inequality', *International Journal of Sociology and Social Policy*, vol 23, no 4/5, pp 159-85.

Theobald, H. (2004) *Entwicklungen der Qualifikationsbedarfe im Gesundheitssektor: Professionalisierungsprozesse in der Physiotherapie und Dentalhygiene im europäischen Vergleich*, Discussion Paper SP I 2004-104, Berlin: Wissenschaftszentrum Berlin für Sozialforschung.

Thiede, M. (2005) 'Information and access to health care: is there a role for trust?', *Social Science and Medicine*, vol 61, pp 1452-62.

Thom, D.H., Hall, M.A. and Pawlson, L.G. (2004) 'Measuring patients' trust in physicians when assessing quality of care', *Health Affairs*, vol 23, no 4, pp 124-32.

Thomas, L., Cullum, N., McColl, E., Rousseau, N., Soutter, J. and Stehen, N. (2002) 'Guidelines in professions allied to medicine', *The Cochrane Library*, issue 2/2002.

Thomson O'Brien, M.A., Oxman, A.D., Davis, D.A., Hynes, R.B., Freemantle, N. and Harvey, R.B. (2002a) 'Audit and feedback: effects on professional practice and health care outcomes', *The Cochrane Library*, issue 2/2002.

Thomson O'Brien, M.A., Freemantle, N., Oxman, A.D., Wolf, F. and Davis, D.A. (2002b) 'Continuing education meetings and workshops: effects on professional practice and health care outcomes', *The Cochrane Library*, issue 2/2002.

Thornley, C. (2003) 'What future for health care assistants: high road or low road?', in C. Davies (ed) *The future health workforce*, Houndmills: Palgrave, pp 143-60.

Thorstendahl, R. and Burrage, M. (eds) (1990) *Knowledge, state and strategy*, London: Sage Publications.

Timmermans, S. and Berg, M. (2003) *The gold standard: The challenge of evidence-based medicine and standardization in health care*, Philadelphia, PA: Temple University Press.

Tophoven, C. (2003) 'Wandel der ambulanten Versorgung', in H. Pfaff, M. Schrappe, K.W. Lauterbach, U. Engelmann and M. Halber (eds) *Gesundheitsversorgung und Disease Management*, Bern: Hans Huber, pp 87-94.

Tovey, P. and Adams, J. (2001) 'Primary care as intersecting social worlds', *Social Science and Medicine*, vol 52, pp 695-706.

Tovey, P., Easthope, G. and Adams, J. (eds) (2004) *The mainstreaming of complementary and alternative medicine: Studies in social context*, London: Routledge.

Turner, B.S. (1992) 'Outline of a theory of citizenship', in C. Mouffe (ed) *Dimensions of radical democracy*, London: Verso, pp 33-62.

Turner, B.S. (1993) 'Contemporary problems in the theory of citizenship', in B.S. Turner (ed) *Citizenship and social theory*, London: Sage Publications, pp 1-18.

Turner, B.S. (1995) *Medical power and social knowledge* (2nd edn), London: Sage Publications.

Turner, B.S. (2004) *The new medical sociology*, New York, NY: W.W. Norton Company.

Ubokudom, S.E. (1998) 'The association between the organization of medical practice and primary care physician attitudes and practice orientation', *Social Science and Medicine*, vol 46, pp 59-71.

Vogel, S. (2004) 'Lernen bringt's', *Niedersächsisches Ärzteblatt*, vol 77, no 10, p 39.

Wagner, M. (1999) 'Medizinalfachberufe im Gesundheitswesen – Wege zur Professionalisierung', *KG-Intern*, vol 2, p 1314.

Weber, M. (1978) *Economy and society* (edited by G. Roth and C. Wittich), Berkeley, CA: University of California Press.

Webster, A. (2002) 'Innovative health technologies and the social: redefining health, medicine and the body', *Current Sociology*, vol 50, no 3, pp 443-57.

Weick, K.E. (1976) 'Educational organizations as loosely coupled systems', *Administrative Science Quarterly*, vol 21, March, pp 1-19.

Wendt, C. (2003) 'Vertrauen in Gesundheitssysteme', *Berliner Journal für Soziologie*, vol 13, no 3, pp 371-93.

Wensing, M., Baker, R., Szecsenyi, J. and Grol, R. (2004) 'Impact of national health care systems on patient evaluations of general practice in Europe', *Health Policy*, vol 68, pp 353-7.

Weselink, D. (2004) 'Ein Physiotherapeut im Management-Team', *Magazin für Physiotherapeuten in Baden-Württemberg*, vol 5, no 10, pp 8-9.

West, C. and Zimmerman, D. (1991) 'Doing gender', in J. Lorber and S.A. Farrell (eds) *The social construction of gender*, Newbury Park, CA: Sage Publications, pp 13-37.

WHO (World Health Organisation) (1981) *Alma Ata 1978: Primary health care*, Geneva: WHO.

WHO (2000) *The world health report 2000 health systems: Improving performance*, Geneva: WHO.

WHO Euro (2001) *Mainstreaming gender equity in health*, Madrid Statement, Copenhagen: WHO Euro.

Williams, S.J. (2003) *Medicine and the body*, London: Sage Publications.

Wilson, A.E. (2000) 'The changing nature of primary health care teams and interprofessional relationship', in P. Tovey (ed) *Contemporary primary care: The challenges of change*, Milton Keynes: Open University Press, pp 43-60.

Witz, A. (1992) *Professions and patriarchy*, London: Routledge.

Wöllenstein, H. (2004) 'Der informierte Patient aus Sicht der Gesetzlichen Krankenversicherung', *Bundesgesundheitsblatt*, vol 47, no 10, pp 941-9.

World Bank (1993) *World developing report: Investing in health*, Oxford: Oxford University Press.

Wrede, S., Benoit, C. and Sandall, J. (2001) 'The state and birth/the state of birth: maternal health policy in three countries', in R. de Vries, C. Benoit, E.R. Teijlingen and S. Wrede (eds) *Birth by design*, New York, NY: Routledge, pp 28-50.

Young, R., Leese, B. and Sibbald, B. (2001) 'Imbalances in the GP labour market in the UK: evidence from a postal survey and interviews with GP leaders', *Work, Employment and Society*, vol 15, no 4, pp 699-719.

ZIPT (Zukunftsinitiative Physiotherapie) (2005) (www.dvmt-maitlandkonzept.de/download/Erklaerung_des_Zukunftsrates.pdf).

ZM (Zahnärztliche Mitteilungen) (2004a) 'Report', vol 94, p 1096.

ZM (2004b) 'Report', vol 94, p 794.

ZVK (Zentralverband Krankengymnastik) (1993a) 'Die Geburt der Krankengymnastik: Ein Beruf setzt sich durch', *Krankengymnastik*, vol 45, pp 1465-9.

ZVK (1993b) 'Historische Entwicklungen der Krankengymnastik', *Krankengymnastik*, vol 45, pp 1317-21.

ZVK Bremen (2003) Unpublished statistics.

ZVK (2004) 'Seperater Nachweis von Physiotherapeuten im Rahmen der Gesundheitspersonalplanung', *Krankengymnastik*, vol 56, pp 1528-9.

ZVK (2005) 'Die Zahl der Physiotherapeuten steigt', *Krankengymnastik*, vol 57, p 137.

Zwarenstein, M. and Bryant, W. (2002) 'Interventions to promote collaboration between nurses and doctors', *The Cochrane Library*, issue 2/2002.

Zwarenstein, M., Reeves, S., Barr, H., Hammick, M., Koppel, I. and Atkins, J. (2002) 'Interprofessional education and health care outcomes', *The Cochrane Library*, issue 2/2002.

Research design of the empirical in-depth study

The empirical in-depth study focuses on actors and processes of change in ambulatory care (research design step III – see Figure i.1). A combination of different methods (triangulation) and different actors and settings provides the best possibility to grasp intersections of interests and different sets of dynamics. A combination of quantitative and qualitative methods is chosen to link representative data on the occupational and organisational structure of office-based physicians and their attitudes on new health policies to specific areas ('switchboards') and groups of actors who 'enable' change. Prior to the main study, numerous expert interviews were conducted with representatives of institutions and associations in health care – including the two health occupations studied here – as well as explorative interviews with physicians. As described previously, the three occupational groups – physicians, physiotherapists and surgery receptionists – represent different positions in the stakeholder arrangement and the health workforce (Chapter Three). Close connections were built up with a number of representatives of institutions and associations during the research process, which enabled me to fill some of the data gaps, and to collect additional material and expert interviews during the research process.

Representatives of an association of SHI physicians, a physicians' chamber and a SHI fund were interviewed in spring 2005 to provide an update as to how the process of merging providers is proceeding. In addition, expert information was collected from consumer representatives in the newly established regulatory boards of the DMPs, the physiotherapists' association and university professors of physiotherapy, as well as surgery receptionists, in order to take the ongoing developments into account. These complex sources of information are included in the analysis, while details are given for the main study (Table A.1).

Following the structure of the German health care system, the focus is on the medical profession. A survey of physicians working in ambulatory care provides an overview of the occupational structure, work arrangements and the profession's attitudes to and appraisal of

Table A.1: Research groups, settings and methods

Research groups and settings	Methods
SHI physicians in one of the western *Länder* of Germany; N=24,526	Survey, mailed questionnaire; N=3,514
Regional provider network, office-based generalists and specialists	Focus group (FG 1)
Quality circles of office-based physicians in different areas of health care, generalists and specialists	Five interviews with group leaders
Regional provider network breast cancer care, specialised physicians and psychologists	Interview with a founding member
Multidisciplinary network of women's health care activists	Focus group (FG 2)
Regional association of physiotherapists	Focus group (FG 3)
Graduates and participants in the first Bachelor studies in physiotherapy	Focus group (FG 4)
Regional association of surgery receptionists	Focus group (FG 5)
Surgery receptionists at the end of a three-year course in an education pilot project	Focus group (FG 6)
Self-help groups of patients with CHD	Focus groups (2) (FG 7, FG 8)
Self-help groups of patients with breast cancer	Focus groups (2) (FG 9, FG 10)
Self-help groups of patients with diabetes	Focus groups (2 diabetes type II; 1 type I) (FG 11, FG 12, FG 13)

the major goals of new health policies. Physicians were surveyed by means of a short written questionnaire, which furnished the following data: (1) appraisal of goals and tools of health policy, for instance, new forms of medical regulation, contracting and the provision of care, EBM, user participation, quality management; (2) implementation level of these goals and tools in the surgery; (3) occupational structure, economic indicators and work arrangements; and (4) individual social-statistical data, such as age and gender.

The area covered by the survey is the total of office-based SHI physicians in North Rhine Westphalia (N=24,526), one of the most innovative regions of the associations of SHI physicians in Germany. The questionnaire was supported and distributed by two associations of SHI physicians, those of North Rhine and Westphalia–Lippe, to all members. The advantage of this method is that it provides access to a very large group and delivers representative data. The response rate, however, was expectedly low overall as the questionnaire was mailed together with lots of routine information of the association. The response rate of 14.3% and a total of 3,514 valid answers lies in the middle to upper range of what could be expected from this way of collecting data. There are no signs of a significant bias with respect to the main indicators, which are used in the statistical analysis of this study; the quota of women is slightly lower in my sample (24%), the quotas of physicians working in general care (48%), and in group practice (29%) are similar to the total of physicians (calculated from personal communication with the cooperating associations and official statistics, see KBV, 2002b); the available data do not allow for an accurate comparison regarding age, but the composition of age groups in my sample does not indicate any significant bias.

This information is complemented by qualitative research on groups from the medical profession and organisational settings that are identified as areas with high dynamics: physicians working in networks, quality circles and members of a multidisciplinary network of women's health care activists. The main areas of interest were similar for all groups and provided the basis for structured focus group discussions or interviews: attitudes towards and implementation of new health policies, especially organisational change; integration of users; cooperation between occupational groups; and tools of bureaucratic regulation and quality management.

In addition to research within the medical profession, focus groups were organised with physiotherapists and surgery receptionists. The research interests necessarily differ according to the different positions of these groups in the system of health care but the focus group discussion is structured according to the general topics. Strategies and attitudes are explored for each occupation in two different groups: the board members and activists of associations, and the 'newcomers'. The latter group is the first to emerge from Bachelor degree courses, recently introduced for physiotherapists, as well as surgery receptionists who were in the process of concluding a three-year education course, which was launched as a pilot project. These groups can be assumed to be key actors to bring change into practice, although on different levels.

The three groups of patients I chose are target groups of DMPs that were in the process of being established, namely, patients in self-help groups for coronary heart disease (CHD), breast cancer and diabetes. The choice of which group of users of health care services to include in this study was made taking the following aspects into account: first, to explore demands on and attitudes of health care providers and health policy from the bottom up, and second, to look at those groups that are currently at the centre of health policy, and will feel the effects of new policies and new models of care most keenly.

The majority of data was collected between March 2003 and

February 2004. Both physicians and patients were surveyed shortly after new directions in health policy CAMe into public discourse and practice. The survey of physicians took place in spring 2003, soon after the announcement of a flexibilisation of contracting between SHI funds and physicians. This was the theme of the Federal Congress of Physicians in February 2003 and subject to strong controversy. Patients were mainly studied in January and February 2004. Starting in 2004, self-payment of patients once again increased and, for the first time, a fixed fee was introduced for every consultation with a specialist that did not follow prior consultation with and referral by a generalist.

Survey data were analysed with SPSS; priority was given to multivariate analysis. The focus group discussions were organised with existing groups, mostly with participants who work together or meet regularly. The only exception to this was the multidisciplinary political network of women's health care activists and the participants in the Bachelor studies for physiotherapy, who mostly knew each other but did not meet regularly in this composition. The discussions were audio-recorded, and the material subsequently transcribed. The additional interviews were carried out either face to face or via telephone, and protocols transcribed. Hermeneutic interpretation was used for the focus groups and interviews.

Index

The political economy of health care
A clinical perspective
Julian Tudor Hart

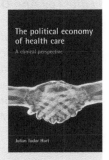

"Health care shaped by market forces and 'commodification' does not deliver services efficiently, let alone equitably. For those who support the principal of universal, equitable access to cost-effective health care, Julian Tudor Hart's radical vision of what is needed will come as a breath of inspiring fresh air." **Sir Iain Chalmers**, Editor, James Lind Library

This is a passionate analysis of the historical development, current state and potential future shape of the National Health Service by distinguished doctor and author, Julian Tudor Hart.

Drawing on many years of clinical experience, Tudor Hart sets out to explore how the NHS might be reconstituted as a humane service for all (rather than a profitable one for the few) and a civilising influence on society as a whole.

Paperback £14.99 US$32.95 **ISBN-10** 1 86134 808 8; **ISBN-13** 978 1 86134 808 1
Hardback £55.00 US$69.95 **ISBN-10** 1 86134 809 6; **ISBN-13** 978 1 86134 809 8
234 x 156mm 336 pages April 2006
Health and Society series

Private complaints and public health
Richard Titmuss on the National
Health Service
*Edited by **Ann Oakley** and **Jonathan Barker***

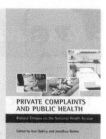

*"With the NHS undergoing the most fundamental change
in its 56 year history, this book is a timely reminder of
important policy dilemmas that we ignore at our peril. This
collection of Titmuss's writings brings together remarkably
prescient commentaries on aspects of health, health care, and
the NHS."* British Medical Journal

Richard Titmuss was one of the twentieth century's foremost social policy
theorists. This accessible Reader is the first compendium of his work on public
health, health promotion and health inequalities.

The book includes commentaries by leading experts in the field making explicit
links between Titmuss's work and key issues of concern in health policy today.

Paperback £19.99 US$36.95 **ISBN-10** 1 86134 560 7; **ISBN-13** 978 1 86134 560 8
Hardback £55.00 US$85.00 **ISBN-10** 1 86134 561 5; **ISBN-13** 978 1 86134 561 5
240 x 172mm 256 pages June 2004
INSPECTION COPY AVAILABLE

Health inequalities and welfare resources
*Edited by **Johan Fritzell** and **Olle Lundberg***

*Foreword by **Lisa Berkman**, Professor of Public Policy,
Harvard University*

How welfare states influence population health and health inequalities has long
been debated but less well tested by empirical research. This book presents new
empirical evidence of the effects of Swedish welfare state structures and policies
on the lives of Swedish citizens.

The discussion, analysis and innovative theoretical approaches developed in the
book have implications for health research and policy beyond Scandinavian
borders.

Paperback £24.99 US$39.95 **ISBN-10** 1 86134 757 X; **ISBN-13** 978 1 86134 757 2
Hardback £55.00 US$90.00 **ISBN-10** 1 86134 758 8; **ISBN-13** 978 1 86134 758 9
234 x 156mm 256 tbc pages November 2006
Health and Society series

Citizens at the centre
Deliberative participation in healthcare decisions
Celia Davies, Margaret Wetherell, and Elizabeth Barnett

Involving citizens in policy decision-making processes – deliberative democracy – has been a central goal of the Labour government since it came to power in 1997. But what happens when members of the public are drawn into unfamiliar debate, with unfamiliar others, in the unfamiliar world of policy making at national level?

Drawing on the lessons from an ethnographic study of a public involvement initiative in the health service – the Citizens Council of NICE (National Institute for Clinical Excellence) – this book sets out to understand the contribution that citizens can realistically be expected to make.

Paperback £23.99 US$42.95 **ISBN-10** 1 86134 802 9; **ISBN-13** 978 1 86134 802 9
Hardback £60.00 US$110.00 **ISBN-10** 1 86134 803 7; **ISBN-13** 978 1 86134 803 6
234 x 156mm 256 tbc pages October 2006

To order copies of this publication or any other Policy Press titles please visit **www.policypress.org.uk** or contact:

In the UK and Europe:
Marston Book Services, PO Box 269,
Abingdon, Oxon, OX14 4YN, UK
Tel: +44 (0)1235 465500
Fax: +44 (0)1235 465556
Email: direct.orders@marston.co.uk

In the USA and Canada:
ISBS, 920 NE 58th Street,
Suite 300, Portland, OR
97213-3786, USA
Tel: +1 800 944 6190
(toll free)
Fax: +1 503 280 8832
Email: info@isbs.com

**In Australia and
New Zealand:**
DA Information Services,
648 Whitehorse Road Mitcham,
Victoria 3132, Australia
Tel: +61 (3) 9210 7777
Fax: +61 (3) 9210 7788
E-mail: service@dadirect.com.au

Citizens at the centre
Deliberative participation in healthcare decisions
Celia Davies, Margaret Wetherell, and Elizabeth Barnett

Printed and bound by CPI Group (UK) Ltd, Croydon, CR0 4YY

27/10/2024

14580558-0003